Andrew Davidson was born in Lambeth in 1959. A former winner of the business writer of the year award, he is a contributing editor of both *Esquire* and *Management Today* magazine, where his monthly interviews with business leaders have appeared for five years. His previous book, *Under the Hammer*, charted the rise of Britain's new breed of television moguls and was shortlisted for the 1993 Krasna-Krautz Award for books on the moving image.

'Well written and fair-minded, *Bloodlines* will tell readers far more about hospital life than any *ER*-style soap opera ... a remarkably accurate impression of what life in a large British hospital is now like'
TLS

Also by Andrew Davidson

Under the Hammer

BLOODLINES

Real Lives in a Great British Hospital

Andrew Davidson

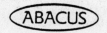

An *Abacus* Book

First published in Great Britain
by Little, Brown and Company 1998
Published by Abacus 1999

A CIP catalogue record for this book
is available from the British Library.

Grateful acknowledgement is made to the following for their kind
permission to reproduce copyright material: Jonathan Cape, an imprint of
Random House UK Ltd for the quotation from *Of Love and Other Demons*
© Gabriel Garcia Marquez, John Berger for the quotation from *A Fortunate
Man*, published by Penguin Books/Granta.

'Don't Look Back in Anger' written by N. Gallagher © Oasis Music/
Creation Songs Ltd/Sony Music Publishing.
Lyrics reproduced by kind permission of the publisher.
'Goodbye Yellow Brick Road' written by Elton John and Bernie Taupin ©
1973, Dick James Music Ltd.
Lyrics reproduced by kind permission of the publisher.

ISBN 0 349 10824 2

Typeset in Minion by
Palimpsest Book Production Limited,
Polmont, Stirlingshire
Printed and bound in Great Britain by
Clays Ltd, St Ives plc.

Abacus
A Division of
Little, Brown and Company (UK)
Brettenham House
Lancaster Place
London WC2E 7EN

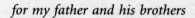

for my father and his brothers

Down in the cellars that run deep beneath the old South Wing at St Thomas' Hospital in London is a curious painting. Daubed roughly on to the crumbling brickwork about three feet off the ground, where the damp cellar corridor meets a T-junction, it depicts a group of startled white rabbits. They gaze lifelessly out of the wall, frozen in time's headlight. A sign next to it explains that it was painted in about 1940. Its intention was to prevent the unwary from walking into the wall during a blackout.

This is a book about one hospital caught at the centre of the recent changes imposed on the National Health Service in London. The events it describes took place between 1994 and 1998. Some names and identifying details have been changed.

REVOLUTION IS A
DAILY EXERCISE

The future will belong to those who have done most for suffering humanity.

Adapted from Louis Pasteur's address to Lord Lister,
Paris 1872

In the more immediate future, early service moves will concentrate on the centralisation of specialities to facilitate the delivery of comprehensive high-quality services and to enable sub-specialities to be co-ordinated from one centre.

Chief executive's report, Guy's and St Thomas'
accounts, 1994/95

1

Meet the doctor. Jim is 33, blond, tall, a little podgy and a keen smoker. Carlos is his patient. Carlos too is a keen smoker, which is why he is being pinned down by two policemen in the Accident & Emergency department at midnight while Jim examines him. Jim smokes filter-tips (in the nurses' tea room). Carlos smokes crack (no one's quite sure where, but the pipe's in his pocket). Right now, Carlos, sweat breaking out over his death-white face, pupils shrunk to pinpricks, looks like he is about to slug someone. His mouth snarls as the shirtsleeved policemen push his elbows back on to the table. His jumper has ridden up, his trousers are open, his flabby pale stomach sags sadly in the harsh white light. Nurses struggle to put pads on his chest and a pulse-clip on one of his fingers. He starts ranting in a guttural foreign language, then grunts some expletives in English.

'Fookin' 'ell! FOOKIN' 'ELL!'

'Stay calm, relax,' says Jim softly. 'We're trying to make sure you are OK, all right?'

'FOOKIN' 'ELL!'

'Can we find someone who speaks his language. What is it, anyway?'

'ARRGGH! FOOKIN' FOOKIN' 'ELL!'

Jim sighs. 'Well, he's got the fucking hell bit OK . . .'

Another night, another customer. Jim, wearing baggy grey trousers and a dancing penguin tie, sits in the tea room and drags on a cigarette. Round the front end of A&E, in the bit the public see, with its wood-effect reception and its Gatwick-style waiting lounge, its pot plants and whispering television, its squeaky clean treatment and resuscitation rooms, the bit where Carlos will later be forcibly restrained, it is all shiny and new, the result of an expensive refurbishment which has turned this particular casualty unit into one of the best-equipped in London. Here, round the back, it's a bit more – how shall we put it? – practical.

Consequently, Jim isn't really in the tea room at all but in a grungy glass booth at the end of it, just big enough for four people. Two air-filters hum. Nicotine seems to drip off the yellowing walls. Outside, large lorries rumble down one of London's main arteries. Inside, a flotilla of coffee cups crowd the tiny table and an old pub ashtray overflows on to the floor. It's the only staff smoking room in the hospital, a quirk ascribed to the nicotine cravings of the old department head.

Jim likes to pop in for a quick one at the start of an evening shift. That's if he can dodge the front desk and anyone who might want his opinion elsewhere. On a night shift like tonight, when the older doctors have gone home, he's in charge from early evening on. As a registrar, he is an experienced qualified doctor, but still about two years away from becoming a consultant, if he's lucky. He has worked in most of the big London hospitals on his way up, and will work in a few more before he's finished. He is, he tells friends, your Joe Average doctor: white, well spoken, middle class, privately educated, non-political. He was even a rugger-bugger as a student. He likes A&E. He likes the buzz and the variety.

He slips on a fresh white coat, standard issue, and clips his name badge to it. The woman who runs the laundry has him pegged for a 42″ chest. Ingeniously, the coats are designed to look ill-fitting, whatever the size. He walks purposefully into the major treatment room, a long, wide room edged with 16 cubicles on three sides, all with trolley-beds and curtains and patients sprawled inside. He looks at the nursing team and smiles to himself, humming a little tune in his head. Who could ask for anything more?

He takes the list of those waiting for treatment from the sister in charge. He smiles, but there is something evasive in his eyes. He has the pudgy, wary face of a young priest already disillusioned with his flock. He's inventing work now, as he doesn't have to see anyone himself; at night he just has to be there to deal with the emergencies and give opinions when needed, to link with the consultants on call and sort out which patient might go where into the maze of the hospital. Jim can wander between major treatment, the kids' unit and the resuscitation room, just checking what's going on. Most of the work is done by the nurses and junior doctors on shift. The junior doctors look much the more pensive, with good reason. Many still feel dangerously out of their depth. For Jim, that's the oddest thing about A&E. Real accidents and emergencies are just the little punctuation points in the long prose of Casualty. Much of the rest is mundane work: people who should have gone elsewhere seen by twenty-somethings barely out of medical school. Yet, after 50 years of the National Health Service, punters still turn up thinking they are going to get better care than from their GP. What they actually get, unless it's a real emergency, is just a bunch of very nervy, very young juniors all over them like a rash. Or, if it's winter, an overrun department too busy to cope. What they become is training fodder. Read that X-ray? I'll try. Squeeze that lump? Ow! Older doctors have their own technical term for it: the sickest seeing the thickest. That's a joke, of course.

Jim, doing his bit, pulls a youth from the queue of patients outside and walks him into a cubicle. The young man is tanned and good-looking, in his early 20s. He has come in with abdominal pain. On the whiteboard chart near the entrance to Major Treatment, the words ABDOM PAIN recur pretty frequently against the cubicle numbers. If you work in Casualty, you see a lot of abdom pain. The young man lifts his T-shirt to show Jim his stomach.

'When did it start?' asks Jim.

'A few days ago,' says the man, looking self-conscious. It got worse when he was at the movies that afternoon, he says. Jim asks him about the film while he prods his stomach. They chat. Jim admires his tan. Jim is wondering whether the man's got a sexually transmitted disease.

'You're a bit of a sun-baby, aren't you?'

Jim is a good doctor. He has got the traditional manner. Slightly patronising, very reassuring, in control and able to put people at their ease. It's what they expect from a doctor, old-style. Jim's consultant thinks he is a very good doctor. People like him. He's calm in an emergency. He doesn't take himself too seriously. When Jim sits down, his trousers ride up to reveal a pair of Mr Greedy socks, which the young man catches with a glance.

Outside the cubicle the evening shift goes about its business. The nurses, trim and taut in blue, pad between cubicles. The young doctors pick their acne and earnestly write up notes at an oblong central station in the middle of the room, heads down, pens scratching, hoping that if they stay there long enough someone might just forget about them. They won't. The system needs doctors. They know what they have to do. The trick is to keep the patients moving, keep pushing them through, get them sorted, get them social services, get them beds, get them out. It's not their problem if the patients bump out a lot of planned surgery further on up the chain. That's just another quirk of the system.

On slow nights like this, Jim yearns for a good trauma case, something juicy, a car crash, a knock-down, a knifing, something really *serious*. It's like being a soldier: he is trained for it, he almost looks forward to it. But most nights, Casualty is just plain dull: geriatrics, winos, junkies, social services cases, abdom pain. This is reality, not the door-slamming, doctor-screaming fiction of popular drama or the hyped-up, heavily edited rush of fly-on-the-wall reports. Television crews, though, do tend to make an evening more interesting. Unless there are any gynaecological cases. Jim hates gynae. Every doctor has his blank spot. Jim's nightmare is a major treatment room full of pregnant women with pre-term bleeding, all the junior doctors asking his opinion, and a TV crew waiting to see what happens. Just the thought gives him a cold shiver.

He would rather leave it to his wife. She's an obstetrician. They make a nice living. He earns around £33,000 a year and has a cosy two-up, two-down in north London. He's got a couple of kids, his wife's on maternity leave and may go part-time soon. Days off for Jim are spent looking after the children, lolling in bed or playing *Theme Hospital* on his computer. Occasionally he dreams of what it would be like to have a cushy little GP's surgery in leafy Surrey, but then he snaps out of it. He'd miss the buzz.

He was always going to be a doctor. His dad was a doctor, his brother, sister and brother-in-law are doctors too. That's what it's like in the old teaching hospitals; in some there are families that have provided doctors for five or six generations. It's clannish and open to accusations of nepotism, but it works. They just keep on coming.

But it's changing too. At St Thomas' there are now far more women doctors, and a big influx of Asian trainees. Of the four or five different students he sees every fortnight, it is unusual to get a majority of white faces. For Jim's generation, it is not a big deal. The Asian doctors are frequently brighter than their white colleagues. Likewise the growing proportion of women: they make better doctors, Jim reasons. More conscientious. Less stuffy. And better at the personal skills, which is what good doctoring is all about. That and memorising huge amounts of information. The rest is mainly pattern recognition, a skill that builds up with experience: once you've seen a number of people with heart failure you can recognise them walking in the door. That's it, really.

He does night shifts and day shifts, and has an 18-month contract at the hospital before he moves to another unit run by a neighbouring trust. Most of his work is dealing with different minor emergencies. He likes it. He did a surgery rotation when he was training, and he couldn't bear the monotony of the routine, operating in the morning, out-patients in the afternoon. Anyway, he hated surgery, cutting into well-looking people, offering themselves voluntarily to the knife. In A&E, it's different. Someone comes in with a stab wound to the chest, the sac round the heart is filling up with blood, it's squashing the organ, you've got to open up the patient and put your finger in the hole. But you can't lose when you make that decision. If the patient dies, everyone says you made the right decision. Surgery is different. It's scary. He resigned, and was told he wouldn't get good references, and he might never work again. Medicine was like that. But he stuck it out, got jobs as a locum in A&E in north London, and look at him now.

The problem with A&E is the stress. Sometimes it's slow, sometimes it isn't. At night, after a long shift with a sudden run of grim accidents – a heart attack followed by a cot death added to three drunken brawls – when you realise that if you don't go home you never will, it's hard to unwind. After a bad one, a stiff whisky and a small temazepam works for most doctors. Out like a light and up fighting fit. But they have to keep it quiet from their families.

Jim often wonders how it all holds together. To run A&E now, you have to be a smart political animal. It supplies the lifeblood of any hospital – sick people – but it is also the most sensitive part of any medical service. It has to be geared up for everything from a splinter in a politician's bottom to a bus-bomb in the Aldwych. Get it wrong and no one lets you forget. Jim watches his boss for clues. His boss, a grey, stooped and eminent consultant, reserves his charm for those who need it, not for outsiders. He prowls the department like an angry old egret, protecting his own. 'I don't need any kind of coverage whatsoever,' Jim's boss tells journalists tersely. 'I can wake up any morning and find my department plastered all over the front pages!'

To run such a department, with its seven-day-a-week, 24-hour-a-day service, with its 100-plus staff and its £5m budget spread between Thomas' and Guy's, you have to be equal parts doctor, manager and Machiavelli. Consider the numbers: it takes 56 nurses, 18 doctors, 14 receptionists, 10 radiographers and 4 nurse practitioners, working in shifts, to keep it open all hours. You have to be prepared to work with what you get and to fight for what you can't. You have to bear the brunt of the winter crises, when the flow slowly puddles at A&E, cut off by the tightening tourniquet of no-beds. That, of course, is something they never actually teach you: how to manage, how to organise, how to turn internal politics to your advantage. Jim's boss doesn't just run two departments: he gives lectures, helps run the speciality nationwide, attends endless councils and cocktail parties, the clink-clink-chatter of every top consultant's evening. And in a hospital like St Thomas' he has conspicuous power: the power of patronage. So many doctors, at some stage or another, go through his department as part of their education. Around 250 junior doctors apply for the 25 senior house officer posts in A&E every year. Even Virginia Bottomley's daughter worked there – another reason for keeping the press out.

Yet the curious thing is that no one has quite worked out yet what makes a good A&E doctor. Most specialists are defined by their diagnostic category, the A&E crew by geography. They have got to be smart, quick, personable and 'diplomatic', a word Jim's boss likes to use in totting up the attributes. The medical key is what they call 'immediate assessment and immediate resuscitation skills in serious trauma and cardiac cases'. That's why the heart of A&E is the resuscitation room. Resus sees the best equipment, the most excitement and a lot of death. Around 100 in the last year alone. Most nights Jim is happy to oversee whatever's going on there. When he's not, he knows it's time to take a holiday. Those are the times when he hears the main bell ring, signifying an ambulance rushing another trauma case in, and just wants to hide under a desk and say, 'I am a tomato, I don't work here.' Those are the times when he couldn't give a toss about the famous old hospital behind him, with its honour boards and veterans and quaint, arcane customs.

2

No one knows now exactly when St Thomas' was founded. There was mention of an infirmary at the Priory of St Mary Overy in 1106 on the site of the first St Thomas' near London Bridge. Renamed in 1215 – after the martyred St Thomas à Becket – it grew as London grew, starting out, like so many medieval hospitals, under the control of the Church. Henry VIII abolished it in 1540, but his son Edward VI reopened it 12 years later, rededicated to St Thomas the Apostle, patron saint of masons and architects. After all, cities need hospitals. It moved to its current location in 1863, redeveloping a barren site on the sandy foreshore of the Thames, a place large enough to accommodate the sudden spread of specialisms in the medical world and St Thomas' new renown as a teaching hospital, sending out its recruits to practise medicine across the globe. The site did have its drawbacks. Between it and Parliament on the opposite bank sluiced the raw sewage that made up most of the river's flow in those days. It is said that some, like Florence Nightingale, the nurse-heroine who trained at the old St Thomas', refused to set foot on the site, so appalled were they at the sheer unsuitability of its position. But, like the city, the hospital continued to grow.

It survived two world wars, it changed from a self-funding, self-determining institution to become part of the National Health Service (NHS) in 1948, it was buried under a new regional structure in the NHS changes of 1973, and nearly bankrupted in the late 1980s when the constant feuding between local politicians and central government was fought out in its

wards and offices. Many expected it to be closed, moved or
at least subsumed under its more efficient-looking rival, Guy's,
just along the South Bank in Bermondsey. Instead, the reverse
happened. In 1993, it returned to relative self-determination as
an equal partner in the newly formed Guy's and St Thomas'
Trust, and two years later it was announced that most of Guy's
acute services were being moved to the Thomas' site. Experts
cited the central position, the traffic flow and the facilities. Staff
at Guy's were horrified and muttered dark threats about cowardly
politicians and Masonic influence. In the old days, it was claimed,
you couldn't even hope to become a consultant at Thomas' unless
you went to a good public school and were a member of the right
Lodge. That influence, despite nearly 50 years of the NHS, had
now extended into Whitehall to save the hospital.

Well, perhaps. Looking at the influx of female and Asian
consultants at the hospital, and the huge range of people that
the institution now employed and treated, many concluded that
such claims were fanciful, but the rumours persisted.

3

A couple of hours later Resus is beginning to fill up. Carlos
has stopped fuck-helling and is sitting on a bed, one of five
against the left-hand wall, surrounded by equipment: drip bags,
defibrillators, gas masks, bottles and boxes, wires and tubes,
none of it really being used. Some how-to posters are taped
to the wall. Jim is rubbing Carlos' back, almost affectionately,
soothing him. The police have gone, a porter has been found
who speaks his language, he has been given a morphine antidote
that brings him down slowly. A young radiographer pulls along
a large ceiling-mounted X-ray machine. Its arm looks like a metal

praying-mantis leg, hovering theateningly over Carlos' chest. The radiologist counts one-two-three and says, 'Hold your breath, breathe in, very good ...' She presses some big buttons on an infra-red handset and it seems as if a little whirr and a click is audible. Carlos hasn't heard any of it.

Jim is worried because he cannot get any information out of the man: what he has taken, where he lives, whether someone can be rung to get him. A blood test shows the oxygen level in the man's blood is low. A three-way conversation via the porter leads nowhere. Carlos claims he only had a couple of beers that night – oh, sure – and won't volunteer any other information.

Jim gets tetchy. 'Tell him I'm not a policeman, I don't want to know about his status as an immigrant, I don't give a shit! I just want to help him! I want to know if he has taken any drugs. I won't tell his family or the police.'

The porter whispers in Carlos' ear. Carlos stares absently into a corner of the room, calm now but still woozy, like a boxer who is struggling to remember how he lost. Eventually a number is found in his wallet and relatives are called. Cases like this piss Jim off. He knows the man will probably discharge himself when he feels like it, and if you don't know what he's taken, you don't know what kind of danger he is in. And anyway, the police are waiting for him outside.

He turns his attention to the next bed, where another man is out cold after an all-day drinking party.

'How's our bottle-of-vodka man?'

The bottle-of-vodka man isn't moving. Another doctor works over him like a mortician, cold with concentration. Jim rings the surgeon on call in the hospital. 'He's got a quarter-inch laceration of the skin. I've stuck my finger in, and I can't feel any fracture ...'

But he's got to be checked out. So many cases in A&E are what anyone else would call self-inflicted. Rule number one for the medical staff: suspend all moral judgement. Jim can't say, 'You shouldn't have got so drunk, you stupid fuckwit,' even if he would like to. His boss has a motto: 'Those who present will be seen.' And so there is no difference in approach for him than for the old lady in cubicle four of Major Treatment earlier, who had been mugged that morning and had two liver-red black eyes to show for it.

And likewise for the boys who are looking for a fight, the girls who get screwed, the gangsters who get knifed and shot and the people who stick bits up each other for fun. All are welcome, and consequently A&E becomes a repository for those with nowhere else to go, the Care in the Community deranged, the old and lost, the lonely. It is also vulnerable to those seeking attention or just some hard drugs to get them through the weekend. Jim can spot those a mile off. They are the ones who know all the pain-killing alternatives, and always have a good reason why they shouldn't take such-and-such. Ah, but the opiate, no, I haven't tried that, it might work . . .

Then there are those who fake fits, and subtle lads with big erections who turn up saying they have got lower stomach pains and can they see a female doctor? There are repeat customers too, hooked on A&E. Behind the receptionist at St Thomas' is a large cupboard. Inside are the files of 'regulars', row upon row on a stack of racks. The receptionists see everything. Eleven-year-old girls asking for morning-after pills. The drunk and the violent. They have to be as battle-hardened as anyone else.

But everyone has their tolerance point, everyone eventually sees something that gets under their skin. For a doctor like Jim there are already little scenes branded on his memory like scars of hurt and humility, scabbing up over the years. The distraught wife whose middle-aged husband has just died in Resus from a heart attack. Outside A&E's smoked glass front window Jim can see the couple's young children waiting, still not knowing. 'I'll tell them,' he says to her, and then wishes he hadn't. Afterwards he goes away and cries for everyone who has died or been hurt or simply passed through his hands, cries for everything he has seen.

At moments like that, the same image always comes back, the

first memory, a 25-year-old woman who had collapsed in the street. Jim was the same age, just training, junior enough to have a few tasks in Resus and a lot of time to watch. They had cut off her clothes, and she lay there naked and dead, beautiful. No one could work out what had happened. An arrhythmia of the heart? Just dropped down dead. Jim learnt early that life hangs by a thread that can so easily be cut. It was unjust and it hurt. Yet he knows he remembers it so well just because she was so pretty.

And then there are the children. The little girl with the bandage round her finger. As he unwinds it a third of her finger just falls sideways off, hanging on a skin hinge, like the top of a Zippo lighter. The look of shock on her face. Shit, bandages can hide a multitude of sins; things just fall apart when you take them off. Like the motorcyclist whose head came off in the helmet. Pop the top of the finger back on, smile a lot, point out that young flesh has remarkable healing properties.

The babies are worse. The cot death brought in still warm. He takes her down to the end section of Resus, in an alcove decorated with a children's alphabet, with its own machines and tubes and masks and posters, all a little smaller or a little differently marked. The bit of Resus that scares everyone. And he works on the baby for half an hour, or 45 minutes, or an hour, with a team of five, or six, standing round, passing equipment, holding machines, but he knows it won't do any good, he just keeps on going because he is saving his own baby, that's her down there. He knows it is hopeless. Eventually he says: 'I'm going to stop now. Anyone disagree?' And the team concurs. He feels like shit. And the mother has probably been watching the whole thing.

He needed a big drink when he got home that night. A really big drink. Maybe a pill. His father used to send them to him when he was fretting over exams. That's doctors for you. Practical people. The funny thing about doctors and drugs, especially illegal ones, is that doctors are really not much different from others of their generation. Older doctors don't take the fashionable drugs, younger ones do. Jim smoked a bit of grass.

He took cocaine once with some mates, but it didn't work for him. He knows doctors who take Ecstasy. He knows doctors who have become alcoholics. He knows doctors who have tried to commit suicide. After all, he reasons, the job is enough to send anyone barmy.

He remembers the woman whose husband died while having sex with her. It was not that unusual. A cardiac arrest. She tells Jim: 'I thought he was coming . . .' Instead he was going. Jim says well, it was horrible for you, but put the boot on the other foot. It's a great way to go. Thinking about it later he wondered if that was the right approach. You build up such a resistance to these kind of situations, you get so used to breezing through death and suffering, you always wonder if you are being desensitised. And yet it is your only defence, your true commitment to professionalism. The worst and best of life. Prometheus and Pandora – words are quick and vain.

4

Tim Matthews slips round the back of the sliding door into the lecture theatre, so quietly that no one notices. A tall, soft man with a chubby face and owlish eyes, he takes a seat by the door, and studies the backs of the heads in front of him. Eight rows of seats, ten across. He does the maths. The room is packed with an assortment of young people: nurses, administrators, clerks. Each with a name tag, a large, handwritten sticky label. Mary. Jo. Kevin. Clare. A few turn round to stare at him, wondering, he's older, in his forties, wearing a double-breasted suit, who is he? Ah, yes, he's the chief executive of Guy's and St Thomas', a man whose £111,000 salary is one of the largest in the health service. Matthews looks up sharply at the ceiling. However often he does it, he never looks terribly at ease speaking to the Marys, Jo's, Kevins and Clares of this world.

The training manager, a tall, determined woman in her early thirties, stands at the front of the auditorium, winding up her conclusion to the first group sessions. This was all her idea: induction day, a chance to meet the other new starters at the Trust, a chance to meet the chief executive and hear a bit about the history of the two old hospitals. She runs an induction day every month, and regularly gets 80 or 90 new bods along, all young, all junior ranks. The Trust, which has over 6,000 staff and is the biggest employer in its particular patch of south London, gets through a lot of new staff every year.

At least with those starting off you get a bit more respect than from the long servers. Both hospitals have had their problems. Everyone is conscious of the bad feeling between the two sites. Passions have run high following the decision to move all acute services to St Thomas'. They nearly exploded at a staff meeting on the Guy's site when the announcement was made. You had to be there to feel it. There were hundreds who couldn't squeeze into the lecture theatre. Flanked by security guards, Matthews pushed his way through to address the angry mob. He had never felt fury like it, and his shy awkwardness just made the crowd seethe. Now the rage is abating, and each new intake of staff is like a pint of fresh blood, clean from the detritus of the past, clear of the antipathies that have dogged the merger day by day. There is at least one up-side to having a high staff turnover.

On the wall behind the training manager eight large sheets of A2 paper have been pinned up, with everyone's name and job listed – the product of the first of her group sessions, the sort of get-to-know-each-other huddles that training professionals love so much. Everyone divided into six groups, placed round a table, given a big felt pen and an outsized piece of paper and told to introduce themselves. Then write down the key bits of information. Get on with it. Fifteen minutes. Some put ages, some put surnames. Now the sheets hang behind her, looking rather

desultorily back at the audience. *Steve Clark, nurse, St Thomas'
A&E, from Australia. Sarah, part-time receptionist, trained to be
a dancer. John, 22, pharmacist, used to work in Essex.* How odd
what some think important and others don't. How inadequate
it all seems, each with his or her own aspirations and experience
and fears, lumped into a name and a job.

The training manager, lithe and bobbed, dressed in an elegant
blue trouser suit and striped jumper, has already warmed the
audience up. She has given a talk on change and motivation, on
how the constant turmoil of merger, relocation and renovation
can abrade everyone's desire to work. She has moved on now
to explaining how the Trust works, handing out photocopied
sheets with the names of the board directors, and a list of the
group services and their heads. Acute medicine, surgery, tertiary
services, clinical services, women and children, dentistry and
dermatology. She runs through the figures. Fourteen hundred
beds; two sites; £300m income; 20,000-plus day cases a year;
20,000-plus elective patients; 30,000-plus non-elective patients.
'Now,' she says loudly, 'everyone see where they fit in?' She raises
her eyebrows quizzically, ironically, like a school-teacher making
jokes for her own benefit. She has perfected a manner pitched
midway between the loudly brash and the knowingly flip. The
new employees, many of them in their early twenties and unused
to this kind of big company welcome, don't quite know what to
make of her.

'OK,' she says, 'I see the chief executive is here. Would you
like to come up front? Let me introduce Tim Matthews.'

Everyone turns to watch as Matthews walks quickly through
the audience to stand beside her by the slide machine. He
looks round and sleek. His suit jacket flops open, revealing
a mauve tie. His greying hair is brushed forward, boyishly,
into a high fringe. A wide grin splits his face above laughing eyes.

'Is that all the build-up I get?' he asks quietly, flirtatiously, just
loud enough for the front rows to hear. He has an attractive

innocence quite at odds with his position. He rocks a bit on his feet, as if trying to appear jovial.

'We'll put the fanfare on later,' says the training manager. She sits down and the audience waits.

'Right, everybody, er, nice to see you all here. OK. Um. How many people here have been working at the Trust for more than a month?'

His manner is tentative, uneasy. A small flurry of hands go up.

'All right. Um. Who expects to be here in, er, two years' time, working for the Trust?'

No one says anything. No hands go up as the audience try to work out what he is asking.

The chief executive's grin begins to look a little forced.

'This is my instant indicator of morale,' he explains softly, not confident enough to say it loudly, as the hands start to go up.

'Good, good,' he says, trying to break the ice. 'A couple of years ago I did this and only one person put their hand up. I thought, oh, shit.'

No one laughs. He goes on: 'Right, um, if you had to describe in one sentence what the Trust was here to do, what do you think that sentence would be?' A tense hush falls on the room.

'To provide quality care for the patients?' says one man tentatively, three rows from the front, visibly reddening as others turn to look at him.

'Very good,' says Matthews. 'But what is distinctive about this hospital? What distinguishes it from hospitals in Woking or Guildford, say?'

No one says anything. Then a voice whispers, 'Teaching?'

'Yes, teaching and research.'

He switches on a new slide. TRUST MISSION flashes up on the screen behind him. It is accompanied by a text: 'To be London's leading university hospital, providing a comprehensive local acute hospital service to people who live and work in London, providing a range of specialised hospital services and working in partnership with the United Medical and Dental Schools (UMDS) to deliver high-quality teaching and research.'

The words, you might think, are the easy bit.

5

Imagine a starfish with half its legs pulled off, or a one-winged bird with a new head. You might then get a sense of the St Thomas' site, its awkward mix of the old and the new, the abruptly finished and the never started. At its heart is the great white cube, North Wing, that dominates the Albert Embankment with a spectacular view of the Houses of Parliament. 'It's a great view,' nod the Thomas' doctors to visiting politicians. 'But we have got to look at you!' cry the MPs. They have a point. Flat roofed, twelve storeys high, clad in white tiles, glistening with sixties functionality, St Thomas' North Wing is reviled by traditionalists but rather admired by others. Designed by hospital specialists Yorke Rosenberg Mardall, opened in 1976 by the Queen, it was the culmination of a twenty-year rebuilding programme aimed at replacing the original Victorian hospital buildings, which had been damaged during the Blitz. The new scheme swept away acres of slum housing and redirected the Lambeth Palace Road. It also, according to some conspiracy theorists, smartly averted the threat of a proposed move for the hospital down to Guildford, something which the consultants, many with lucrative private practices based in London, were keen to avoid.

Phase one of the redevelopment was completed in 1966, when East Wing, a T-shaped tower rising above a sprawling Accident & Emergency centre, was opened. Phase two consisted of the cuboid North Wing, as well as a smaller treatment block, now known as the Lambeth Wing. There was also a residential block for staff (Gassiot House), an underground car park and an ornamental garden by Westminster Bridge. Phase three, the rebuilding of South Wing, the last remants of St Thomas' Victorian riverside frontage, into two more white cubes, never happened. There were rumours at the time that someone got the measurements wrong and the new blocks would never have fitted in the site anyway.

In some ways, what was left was an effective use of space (North Wing and Lambeth Wing offered 11 hectares of floorspace on around 3.6 hectares of ground), but for those who worked there the new layout gave the site a curious feeling of dribbling away down the Lambeth Palace Road. You simply decreased in importance the further away you were from the new block. It was immediately less communal and enjoyable as well. Replacing an old Victorian system of low buildings joined by long corridors with a squat up-down tower meant you just didn't meet as many colleagues as you used to, tramping on long walks between departments and patients. Everyone was going everywhere in lifts. Suddenly departments felt cut off. Nor did it ever democratise the old regime. The consultants kept their own little dining room off Central Hall, and the beautiful old Governors' Hall, complete with its large portrait of Edward VI, the boy who reopened the hospital after his father had closed it, was eventually refurbished and kept for sherry parties and Lodge meetings. Old and new co-existed. The structures appeared to change but the pattern remained the same.

So St Thomas' was left with a hotch-potch, a web of corridors and access points that were a security nightmare, a front at the back, a reception at the side, an old Central Hall that was no longer at the centre, a garden too close to the traffic and a jumble of portakabins, car parks, and builders' mess in the middle. It possessed neither the elegant calm of Guy's Hospital's old cloisters nor the airy, upward, glassy sweep of the new Chelsea & Westminster. Just the functionality of those white tiles which doctors used to hate so much. White urinal tiles; very apt for a service that many felt was always being pissed on by their friends across the river.

But it was built with idealism. The views from North Wing, designed primarily as a ward block with patients' beds by the windows and managers' offices in the centre, were part of the patient therapy. Just looking at that sweep of London, the Houses of Parliament, the Thames, St Paul's dome in the distance, lifted the heart. North Wing and the adjacent, lower-slung Lambeth Wing, the treatment block, cost around £9 million. The central lifts may have been too small and too few, the plaster may have started dropping off the walls as soon as it was opened, the out-patients waiting rooms may have been the wrong size, but the main spaces were wide and bright, and money was set aside by the hospital's Special Trustees, guardians of the immense wealth that the institution had drawn in over the centuries, for the purchase of the right kind of art: contemporary, non-representational works by the likes of Eduardo Paolozzi (lift lobby) and Patrick Caulfield (X-ray department). The Tate Gallery even lent a Naum Gabo fountain (which broke down repeatedly and cost a small fortune to run) for the garden. The new St Thomas' was to be a place – as the original architects' brief, written by the hospital governors, stated – where 'the art of healing and the art of teaching should proceed hand-in-hand', where its 'third function' of research could be given greater emphasis than ever before, and where the training of 'character' was to be as important as the training of minds. 'Any university fails when it neglects to create an environment in which its students can receive some measure of inspiration from being in a place where people are devoted to the pursuit of the sciences and the arts for their own sake.' The governors wanted it all, and it is hardly surprising that, in reaching for the stars, they got stuck a little way up in a cloudbank. Most of the medical staff were just happy if everything worked.

6

The surgery list starts at 1.30 sharp. The locker room for changing is a good two-minute walk from the operating theatres. Tony Young, surgeon and medical director, the hospital's most senior doctor, is still struggling to get his locker door open. He knows from experience that when the key sticks, you have to be careful not to slice your finger open on the metal fitting by forcing it too hard. He tries another gentle turn; it gives reluctantly, and the long locker door yawns open.

He slips off his shoes, shirt and trousers, briskly folds the latter on a hanger and locks the lot inside. He puts on a pair of turquoise elasticated-waist trousers and a turquoise shift top, slips a turquoise tie-back hat over his grey-white curls, and, after making a little pinched-bend for his distinguished nose in the metal beneath the thin fabric, attaches a turquoise mask. It has two ties, one above the head and one behind the neck. He simply lets it hang loose around his neck, slips a pair of white clogs on his feet and rubs his hands in readiness. He makes the long walk down two corridors on his own.

In the operating theatre his team waits, chatting idly in groups, whispering about love or lunch or money, all resplendent in turquoise, already masked and hatted like a bandit pyjama gang looking for a stick-up. The theatre is long and wide, with three separate anterooms: scrubbing up, anaesthetics and laying out. Twelve large striplights divide the ceiling, and large multi-bulbed operating lights hang over the central table. In such light every fabric wrinkle, every crease and fold of flesh is visible.

The mood quietens slightly when the medical director walks in. He has a patrician gravitas that goes with his Roman emperor looks: strong nose, thinning hair, blue eyes – a certain humour in his majesty. He lathers his hands at the long, low steel sink in the scrubbing-up room, taking care to choose the pink disinfectant rather than the brown one, then ties on a wide green operating gown. His long hands look white and baby-soft as he snaps a pair of latex gloves around them. Behind him, the patient has appeared as if by magic on the table. At one end, the anaesthetist holds court with his machines. At the other, a scrub nurse wheels over a trolley of scalpels, scissors and clamps. In a corner of the room, another nurse enters the details of the operation into the theatre computer: time scheduled, estimated case length, time admitted. The data list appears endless.

'Right,' says Young, taking up his position by the patient's left side, wiping at the brown antiseptic on the exposed abdomen. He bends slightly and concentrates, deep in thought. He could be thinking about medicine, or management, or both.

7

A patient recovering from an appendix operation runs out of his North Wing ward on the eleventh floor in the middle of the night, wearing only his dressing gown. The hospital is quiet, asleep, ticking over till morning. The alarm is raised. Security staff find the dressing gown two floors down, but no sign of the man. Eventually the police are called in with tracker dogs. A missing-persons alert is put out. No one sees him. The patient is found four weeks later, dead, crouched behind ducting pipes in a machine room on the third floor.

These things happen in a big hospital. The Trust handles over 20,000 day cases, more than 20,000 elective cases, over 30,000 emergency admissions. Most go home happy patients – and then this. The man's widow is outraged and demands a government inquiry. She doesn't get one. Newspapers leap on the story. An internal inquiry concludes that more effort must be made to prevent access to service areas.

The facilities men who spotted his body reckon that a couple of weeks later they might never have found him at all. His body had begun to dry out, and would soon have stopped smelling. There he would have stayed, wrapped in eternal paralysis, right at the heart of the hospital. Cheating time.

8

No one would wish merging two famous old hospitals on any manager, especially two institutions that had been in acrimonious competition for the last decade. But Matthews had wanted the job, and got it. People said he was a brilliant consensus manager. Nervous public speaker, awkward presence, a bit diffident, but a shrewd manipulator and perfect for a position which required a sensitive touch and certain sponge-like qualities. He was warm and friendly, and liked the good things in life – he even listed champagne drinking as a hobby in his Who's Who entry – and he was sharp and witty, too, when he wanted to be. 'Is Hunt's House listed?' someone had asked him after his induction day speech to joiners. Hunt's House is a decrepit old block scheduled for redevelopment, running through the centre of the Guy's site. 'Listed?' he said with that wide smile. 'More like listing!' NHS chief executives, who were normally rather grey men, were not supposed to make jokes like that. What would the new staff make of it?

He was born in Kent, brought up in Devon. His father had worked in the cement industry, his mother had been a teacher.

It was odd how many people you found in the hospital who had one or other parent as a teacher – it must be the public-service ethic. He was a bright boy, did well at Plymouth College, won a place at Cambridge at the start of the seventies, got a 2:1 reading history at Peterhouse, the most right wing college you could choose. Like so many bright boys then, he opted for the civil service. It was a three-stage process to get into the Department of Health and Social Security: verbal reasoning exams, IQ tests, board interviews, that kind of thing. He loved that kind of thing, and excelled.

Why health? He wasn't sure himself, when asked. He had worked as a porter at Addenbrooke's for holiday cash when he was a student. He was probably one of the few chief executives to have seen hospitals from both ends, as it were. Most chief executives had been in hospital management all their lives. He hadn't. Maybe he was interested in health. It certainly looked that way when, as a junior civil servant, he worked on reviews of hospital services in central London and plugged away at the financial structure of the NHS. By the 1980s, a new government had come in under Margaret Thatcher, offering a rather aggressive approach to manpower in the civil service. Gone were the cosy days under successive Labour and Conservative administrations when everyone agreed the civil service had a job to do. Suddenly, promotion prospects reduced dramatically. Matthews knew people working in health authorities; a job came up in central London; he chatted to the guy who was district administrator; he was asked if he was interested. 'Well, actually, funny you should say that. I am,' he replied. He joined as director of planning.

Later he became one of three general managers responsible for a certain central London hospital. As soon as he got in, the health authority told him to close the A&E as it wanted to put the service into another hospital half a mile away. That's hospital management for you. The staff were furious, but he handled it and stayed there three years. Then he wanted his own hospital to run, something bigger, something meatier. He wanted to be chief executive of a district. Despite his diffident exterior, Matthews was an ambitious man.

He looked at a lot of jobs around London. He didn't really want to shift his family. Then a job came up that he liked the sound of, general manager of a health authority in Kent. He took it and reverse-commuted down the A20. It was great – the authority was smaller and less complex than the set-up in central London, but much broader, and with a different feel. County politics were somewhat easier to handle than Camden politics. No surprise there, of course. And when the next round of health-service reforms came in, he was grateful to be in a more protected environment, not sitting in central London, sweating, don't panic, don't panic.

They were strange reforms, launched by Ken Clarke with a big, glitzy PR campaign, but actually containing few details, just some headline objectives. Then working parties were set up to try and decide how to reach those objectives. He was invited on to the working party looking at Project 26. He never knew why it was called Project 26. It sounded faintly Orwellian, like Room 101. It was a mysteriously anonymous title for something which was to become so infamous. It was set up to examine the purchasing arrangements in the new split between purchasers and providers. Interesting times.

But he missed the buzz of the big London teaching hospitals, the arrogant charm of the great doctors, the sniff of the media hounds on his trail. Then one day he saw the chief executive's job at St Thomas' advertised in the *Health Service Journal*. He thought about it. St Thomas' was one of the most famous hospitals in Britain, bang opposite the Houses of Parliament, with a catchment area that seemed to stretch from Peckham to Plymouth. Running it was one of the top health jobs in Britain. He knew it was what he wanted, but should he wait? Right now, it looked a lame duck, it had nearly gone bust when under local-authority control in the NHS financial crisis of 1988–89.

By 1990 no one even knew if the hospital was going to survive. It had had its trust application refused, while down the road its sister hospital, Guy's – they shared the same medical school – was a flagship for the government health-service reforms. To cap it all, internally it was a mess. The Government had sent an ex-British Rail chairman in to sort out the rancour. The doctors, many of whom were world-class, but who had the reputation for being among the snottiest in the NHS (old medical joke: why are St Thomas' doctors all uncircumcised? Because you have to be a complete prick to work there), were exasperated with both politicians and management. Then there were all the old rumours about the Masonic influence. It was no secret. There was even a display of Masonic regalia in the hospital's Governor's Hall, for God's sake. All in all, if you were going to choose a really tough job to leap into, being boss of St Thomas' looked about as bad as you could get, especially if you weren't a pinny-wearer. Matthews wasn't, but he was an ambitious man.

He got the job. Then the Government announced the Tomlinson enquiry into London hospital services. Everyone presumed closure was on the cards. St Thomas' was a sitting duck. Every week it felt as if the London *Evening Standard* was writing the same story: St Thomas' to go, St Thomas' for the axe. Suddenly the chief executive began to feel the pressure from all sides, from the health authority, from the emerging purchasers. Let's rationalise services in south London. Shouldn't you be going along with it? You cannot waste money fighting for survival. No, no, no. Absolutely not.

He talked with the senior doctors and all the old management team. They agreed: they could roll over, kick 800 years of history into the Thames, and look for jobs elsewhere. Or they could fight. And not just fight in a timid, gentlemanly way, but really fight, no-holds-barred, up-front PR, to save the hospital. Let's do it, he said. You're right, said the managers. Completely right, said the doctors. And I've a suggestion, added the chairman. I know just what we need. So, much to the Government's horror, and the health department's fury, and everyone outside St Thomas' dismay, the chief executive pulled funds out of the Special Trustees, that repository of huge wealth given to the hospital over the years, and hired Sir Tim Bell, Margaret Thatcher's favourite public-relations expert.

That got the issue on the *Today* programme. The chief executive was grilled: why are you wasting money given to the hospital by grateful patients? Shouldn't it be spent on toys for the children's ward, or tellies for the nurses, or new gardens for the sick and disabled? But, he replied, there will be no wards or nurses or patients if the hospital goes. He had a strategy, and he stuck to it. If the hospital appeared loud and self-confident and successful, if it was prepared to stand up for itself, it would be less easy for others to chip away at it. And most importantly, the doctors backed him up. Within any clinical community there are those who watch, and the few who get active. This time, they all got active; they lined up right alongside him. They had the best contacts, all the VIPs they had ever treated, and they used them, ringing them up, sending out information packs, reminding them of what the hospital had done for them. It was unashamed campaigning, the pulling together of nearly 50 years' experience of internal NHS politics. There was no suggestion of merger then, just a fight for survival.

In fact, everyone assumed that the Tomlinson enquiry would simply choose to close either St Thomas' or Guy's. There had to be some rationalisation of services in south London in order to provide better community-based primary care (which had always been neglected in the capital). Lewisham and King's hospitals could not be closed as they really did have their own populations to serve. But St Thomas' and Guy's, too such big, expensive hospitals just a mile apart, serving the same area? In the end, everyone underestimated politicians' love of a fudge. Not closure – that might lose votes – but merger became the preferred option. The medical schools had been put together in an earlier round of rationalisations; suddenly it seemed logical that the hospitals should follow suit. After all, for hundreds of years they had operated virtually as twins, sharing adjacent sites off St Thomas' Street near London Bridge. Then St Thomas' had moved to the Albert Embankment. Now the twins could have a friendly reunion. Tomlinson recommended merger in November 1992. The Government told the respective hospital managers: 'Get on with it. And have some ideas in place as to how you are going to do it by April 1993.'

So, after having been the most intense rivals, the teams at St Thomas' and Guy's had to sit down together and draw up a merger plan. It was totally bizarre, but that's hospital management for you. For a start, both hospitals were run with different priorities. At St Thomas', long-serving NHS consultants, who devoted a sizeable amount of time to their private practices, tended to call the shots. At Guy's, which prided itself on its academic excellence, medical research held sway. But both sides agreed a moratorium on conflict, and put in place 'processes'. Looking back, of course, Matthews should have realised that this was just the easy bit, because it was only about merging management. They hadn't even started on the clinical side. But a chairman of the new would-be Trust was appointed in January, then a handful of non-executive directors were brought in, and in February, the two chief executives were allowed to interview for the one boss's job. Up until then, both management teams had worked together not knowing which boss would be chosen, or even if an outsider would be appointed. Indeed, an outsider would have been a smart choice, given the lingering animosity between the two sites. But in fact, everyone assumed that Peter Griffiths, the chief executive of Guy's, would get it: he was high up in the NHS hierarchy, he had good contacts, he was an inspirational leader, and he looked the man for the part. But he didn't get it. Perhaps he was overconfident. Perhaps he didn't realise how subtly Matthews would campaign for the job. Perhaps, given Guy's dominant influence in the medical school, it was felt that some balance was needed.

On 22 February 1993, the medical world woke up to a surprise. The chief executive of St Thomas' had got the job. Some were stunned. How could the Thomas' man have got it? How could the boss of a huge hospital that only a few years back had been on its knees, bankrupt and discredited, have been given the top slot in what would be the biggest NHS trust in Britain? What was worse, St Thomas' had campaigned so aggressively. Wasn't it all a vindication of bad behaviour? How could that be condoned, or even rewarded? On the Guy's site, the senior medical staff couldn't believe it. Guy's had been the first hospital trust, it had fought the good fight for the Government in its health-service reforms, it had always produced much better medical research than its rival, it hadn't campaigned overtly, it had been well behaved, it was in the middle of putting up a hugely expensive new building (the size, as they kept pointing out, of an average district general hospital). And now this?

In fact, it wasn't so strange a decision. Matthews had proved his financial acumen – he had staunched the haemorrhaging of cash out of St Thomas' and bolstered revenue – and he had the voluble support of his doctors, which Griffiths probably hadn't. But when his appointment was followed by the announcement that eventually all acute services, including A&E, would be moved to the St Thomas' site, the staff at Guy's were bewildered and outraged. Acute services were the glitz of being a doctor: the emergencies, the tough stuff. Not just chopping off haemorrhoids, going, 'Oh, it's Monday, it must be Mr Jones at nine and Mrs Smith at ten.' But the brain-stretching, sweat-dripping, nerve-crunching end of medicine, the stuff they watch on *ER* and *Casualty*, and tut-tut over but secretly adore. Striding down the corridor in your theatre greens. It's an emergency! Out of the way! It's OK, the doctor's coming! That's what they'd trained for. That's what got their colleagues talking at dinners and cocktail parties all over London. And not just emergencies, but life-threatening diseases, hideous deformations, crumbling bones and poxy lungs. Patients' lives just hanging on the edge in Intensive Care. Fascinating cases to fuel their research. The chance for stardom.

Not haemorrhoids at nine.

Of course, it didn't seem a big deal to a lot of people outside the medical world. To many of the staff at St Thomas', though, it was like winning the Lottery. But the hospital absorbed success as easily as it shrugged off failure. It had its own way of doing things.

9

In the X-ray department a visitor waits for the senior consultant. He stands in the consultant's tiny office, studying the small framed photo of the 1971 Arsenal Double-winning team that hangs on the wall. Next to it is a print of the original Victorian design for St Thomas', with its sweep of turrets, balconies and corridors abutting the Thames. The consultant is down the corridor, giving advice to a colleague, their conversation faintly audible through the open door. The visitor moves his weight from his left foot to his right, and sucks in his cheeks.

The consultant, a radiologist, is one of the hospital's great men. Slightly round-shouldered and grey-haired, with a domed head and a beaky nose, he looks as if he has spent a lifetime hunched over vast metal machines, cogitating and calibrating. Then he opens his mouth, and you realise his reputation is underscored with a blunt northern humour. Unusually for his generation of Thomas' consultants, he didn't train at the hospital but across the river at Bart's, the only London hospital reputed to be snottier and more inward-looking than Thomas'. He admits it himself with a laugh – in his first year at Bart's, 23 out of 25 students had relatives working at the hospital. Virtually all went to public schools. He himself went to grammar school in Sheffield, yet it never held him back in the London medical world. The medical world could be fiercely meritocratic when it wanted to be.

'Hello, how are you doing, distinguished son of a distinguished father?' he says, greeting his visitor with his customary wide smile and all-too-knowing flattery. He has a way of sticking his chin out as he grins, staring at his interlocutor along his nose, always with a twinkle in his eye. The visitor, who doesn't know him well, is embarrassed, but suspects the consultant can cut the oil with some vinegar when he wants. He has that look. He was a good friend of the visitor's father, who was also a Thomas' consultant. 'He was a great man,' says the radiologist. 'No side to him whatsoever.' He explains that it has been a difficult fortnight for him. His own father has just died, and he has been up north to sort out his dad's papers. There, in a drawer, he found all of his old school reports. Funny what your parents keep, isn't it? he says. Elsewhere, he's dug up some photos, including one of him with his friend, the visitor's father, at Ascot in 1989, with their wives. A couple of swells. 'We look a picture in that,' he says. He pauses. A small frisson passes between them in that tiny room, a shiver of loss and regret for fathers and friends everywhere.

He has promised to show his visitor around the department, one of the busiest and best equipped of its kind in Britain. They set off at a lope, down corridors, through rooms, round in a wide circuit. The department is huge. Nearly every patient who comes into hospital goes through it, or gives it work, at some time. The consultant runs through all the equipment and what it does: X-rays, ultrasound, CT scans, MRI scans, angiography. It seems endless. How much does that cost? asks the visitor, confronted with another large metallic white machine. Around a million, says the consultant. And this? A million and a half, probably. And all this? They are standing in what looks like a control room, where another doctor, in green trousers and top, is drying his hands. The equipment in the adjoining room looks even vaster than elsewhere. What do you think? the consultant asks him. One and a half, maybe two million, smiles the man.

These machines that see through your skin, cut photographic slices out of your body, follow this fluid and that, each cost a small fortune to buy and run but are now essential, he explains. They are the key diagnostic tools in the hospital. There is even one in the basement, he continues, wagging his finger, that pinpoints your cancer. They give you a substance, it goes into the bloodstream, the machine throws up a whole body picture, and the spots which glow are where the cancer is. It is called the Positron Emission Tomography centre. Tomography? Later the visitor looks it up: 'a technique of using X-rays to create an image of a specific thin layer through the body', says the dictionary. Like so much of the 20th-century medical vocabulary, it means nothing at all to outsiders. The visitor saw the sign on the way in: PET centre in basement. He had wondered then if it was where the doctors left their dogs.

The visitor is now boggled. How does a doctor keep up with all the changes in technology? How does a hospital afford it? Hospitals don't, says the consultant. Much of the equipment at Thomas' is bought with the help of the hospital's Special Trustees. They are the stewards of the hospital's own private cash mountain, the result of eight centuries'-worth of endowments and donations. Like an Oxbridge college, St Thomas' has farms in East Anglia, property in London, fantastically valuable artworks and over £100 million pounds on the Stock Exchange. It is not something it shouts about. Much of the interest from that wealth, astutely ring-fenced from the politicians over the years, is dispersed in the form of grants for medical research and donations towards new equipment.

At this point the visitor is beginning to see how the links between the medical and the Medici (pills on their coats of arms, indeed) are as apt as ever. The consultant tilts his head and peers beadily at his guest. He smiles cynically. 'People come into this fabulous hospital: they see that it's clean, it's got lovely pictures on the wall and state-of-the-art equipment. They say, "Thank you, NHS!" But a lot of it is there simply because the Trustees have given it.' How long did it take King's College Hospital to get a CT scanner? he asks. His visitor shrugs. 'I don't know, how long?' They didn't get it till 1987, or 1988. Tell me any comparable-sized hospital in America that didn't get one ten years earlier, says the consultant. King's had to raise the money rattling cans around pubs in south London. But Thomas' got its scanner in 1977 because its Trustees chose to pay for it. It has always been a lucky hospital that way. Without its Trustees, he says, this department, at the very core of the hospital, would be pretty bare. Without its Trustees, the visitor hears him mutter as they walk on, he would have left a long time ago.

They move from room to room, corridor to corridor, across the lino floors. The department, like so many others, is a labyrinth, windowless, striplit and starkly grey, each room, each corridor, much like any other. Here, though, there is no smell, no chemical tinge or sniff of fear like in the wards. Here, of course, there are relatively few patients. Just the quiet bustle of technicians working machines, and the odd pocket of contemplation, as white-coated specialists study X-rays clipped up on light boxes. They enter one such room. A pretty female doctor sits with a student either side of her, studying an X-ray on the box in front of them. She smiles at the consultant. He introduces her to the visitor. Each is defined by a parent: she is the daughter of so-and-so, a Thomas' man, and he, of course, is the son of such-and-such, also, of course, a Thomas' man. It is the same in the room adjacent to the MRI scanner. Another woman doctor sits poring over the screens. In front of her, through a small window, the great grey whale of the machine gapes darkly. Behind her, a male nurse and a colleague sit, playing with a baby in a pram. 'And this is . . .' starts the consultant, 'who is the daughter-in law of . . .' he continues, 'who is of course one of our most famous . . .' The visitor is amused. Every doctor is the son or daughter of someone else who works here, it seems. 'I hope you can see that it's still a family business,' says the consultant, winking, when the two of them are alone again. The visitor, whose own father wanted him to go into medicine, sees now what he has missed.

10

'YER FUCK! YER FUCKING FUCK!'

Two shirtsleeved policemen have brought a youth into A&E. He is bleeding from his shaven head, he has lost his shirt and his abuse is splenetic. The veins tighten and protrude in his chest as he struggles to break out of their grip.

'GET YER FUCKING HANDS OFF ME, RIGHT? GET YER FUCKING HANDS OFF ME!'

'Come on, calm down.'

'YER FUCK!'

The sister on duty tells the policemen to let go. She talks quietly into the boy's ear. He pants nervously, shaking slightly, like a broken horse.

11

And then there's the politics. Jim is on the phone in A&E, talking to a urology consultant. It is midnight. A baby has been brought in with a dick like torn radish, bleeding heavily after a botched circumcision. The parents are frantic. 'Look! Look! CAN'T YOU HELP HIM!' implores the father. The mother just cries.

The urology registrar, on call somewhere in the huge hospital behind, can't be found. Either his aircall batteries are flat, or he hasn't got it with him, or he's not where he should be, or . . . Jim has woken the registrar's boss, asleep at home. Jim wants to say, 'Look, this kid needs a urology operation, he's exsanguinating, I've got a nurse holding his willy and we've got to do something!' but he's politer than that. You have to be careful who you pick fights with; you might want favours later.

Usually it's just placing patients. Getting the old lady with the broken arm a bed because she has no one to look after her at home. Orthopaedics don't want her because the arm will mend itself. Care of the Elderly never have any beds available. Jim can beg and wheedle. If it's night-time he can ring his boss at home. Or if he's feeling bolshy he can ring someone else's boss because they won't play ball. Most doctors are OK, but there's always one Neanderthal wherever you work who will never take your patients.

It's all done on the phone. A&E is like a transit camp, a striplit and disinfected Ellis Island, sorting out the arrivals, pushing some through to the hospital, holding others longer, rejecting a few who are just wasting everyone's time. The odd thing is that Jim knows little about what goes on in St Thomas' itself, with its statues and alumni lists, its old Governors' Hall and panelled consultants' dining room, its legendary cliques of Masons, misogynists and toffs. A&E is its own little world, vital to but somehow apart from the very institution for which it is often the only public face. It is the one bit you can walk into and be seen without appointment. It is also the one bit you can work in and never walk through the hospital at all.

And right now, in the nineties, as every A&E doctor knows, it is not a bad place to work. Sure, some units are being closed as policy insists on fewer, bigger A&E departments. But more people are using A&E, more money is going into it, and most doctors acknowledge that bigger departments mean better facilities, better expertise and better care. It won't affect the number of doctors needed either. The specialism only got consultant status in the seventies. Younger doctors like Jim could do the arithmetic: around 250 A&E departments in England and Wales, around 300 A&E consultants. Most of the junior doctors who train in A&E are just doing it for the experience, passing through. Room for a lot more consultants. Not too many worries on the future employment front, then. Jim has already done his specialist exam and is a Fellow of the Royal College of Surgeons (Edinburgh). There may not be much opportunity for private work on top, but writing the odd report for the police on an assault victim – £24 a shot – keeps him in fag money.

Jim punches the keyboard at a computer in the Major Treatment room. After the screen-savers – laughable aphorisms like *The Joys Of Spring* and *May the Sun Always Shine Upon You* – scroll past, the numbers come up. It is May. Patient number 30,000-and-something has just gone through. Three years ago St Thomas' A&E handled about 65,000. This year it will near 90,000. Soon it will be 100,000. Where are they all coming from? Why are they coming? Do the ones that aren't accidents and aren't emergencies think they are getting a better service than seeing their GP? The abdom pains. The headaches. The itches.

Jim is called to a cubicle in Major Treatment by a senior house officer who wants his verdict on a skin problem. Inside the cubicle, behind a curtain, a short, shy woman in her twenties unbuttons the top of her shirt to show Jim a growing red stain across her neck and chest. Hmm, goes Jim. Hmm, goes the SHO. She says it started before the weekend. Hmm, they go. She couldn't get an appointment with her GP till next Friday. Take one of these, we'll fix you up with an appointment at dermatology, says Jim. There are, Jim says to himself, lots of GPs in central London he wouldn't bother going to see either.

And maybe people just worry more nowadays too. Governments can't spend millions on health-education campaigns, extolling the virtues of preventing rather than curing, and not expect a knock-on effect. They cannot keep squeezing hospitals to be more efficient, kicking patients out quicker and pushing those with mental disorders on to the street, without expecting some kind of bounce-back. And then there is always more a hospital can do for people: it is the march of technology. The only certainty is that you cannot control what's coming through the door. You could divert it, of course, running primary-care emergency centres staffed by GPs next to A&E. It's one idea. No one is that sure how it would work, though.

What would help is if the politicians would stop buggering around with the system. Jim, like the majority of doctors, is not a political animal. He doesn't like working ludicrous hours as a junior doctor, spending every other night on call; he wouldn't wish that on his worst enemy. But now it seems to him that junior doctors just clock on and clock off, with little commitment. More importantly, no one looks as if they are having fun any more. It is all too busy, too earnest. What's the point in having huge hospitals if everyone is miserable? There is no time for the traditional medical stuff: playing football in the corridor with the nurses while the rest of the hospital sleeps, or seeing how many people you can get into a cupboard. Quite a lot, if you're up for it.

12

Why do we have big hospitals? There is a simple, logical answer – they are an efficient concentration of resources and expertise – but that is constantly undermined by everyday observation, historical analysis and the occasional reasoned argument. We have big hospitals because originally, in medieval days, those who ran cities needed a way to get the sick poor off the streets. We have big hospitals because 200 years ago the Industrial Revolution concentrated the workforce in such a way, creating an upsurge in disease and injury, that the back-street quacks and travelling medics couldn't cope. We have big hospitals because, 100 or so years ago, doctors realised that they could be a useful place in which to raise their profiles and generate more cash for their private practices. We have big hospitals because, 50 or so years ago, they were deemed to be one of the bedrocks of the new British welfare state.

None of which, of course, militates against them being an efficient concentration of resources and expertise, but experience says they are not. Now, according to some who work in them, a succession of politician-led changes have turned the larger teaching hospitals into huge, impersonal illness factories, in which the patients are just fodder for the ravenous medical schools that run them – human guinea pigs for the students and academic researchers to learn on. These institutions rarely serve their local communities well, and are neither as humane nor as enjoyable to work in as they used to be, especially since the emphasis on primary care means that patients have to be a lot sicker to get into hospital.

'It has all changed,' moans a senior surgeon. 'The attitudes have changed, the illnesses have changed. The technology that we chuck at the patients has changed. The length of stay in hospital has changed. Patients' expectations and doctors' expectations and nurses' expectations have changed. The hours of duty have changed. You name it, it has changed, in the last 20 years. In the old days you felt you were working as part of an organisation to a particular end, the pace of everything was slower and the patients weren't so hugely sick. There was less pressure, more sense of community and more of a sense of ownership. Nowadays, four-fifths of the patients you are looking after you have never seen before . . .' He wipes his hand through his sparse hair, wondering why even discussing the bald facts makes him feel so powerless.

13

'Ready?' says Young to his team.

No one answers. He is still standing, masked, hatted, gowned, gloved and clogged (natty little white numbers with his initials on the heels), waiting to make the first cut.

The anaesthetist, the registrar, the two nurses and the trio of students all follow the knife. It is held above a large expanse of marble-smooth belly, streaked with iodine-based antiseptic and bordered by green surgical drapes. The belly breathes slowly, in time with the faint phtt-pok of the operating theatre ventilator, the only sound audible, phtt-poking away behind the little green screen that separates the patient's head from the exposed abdomen.

'OK, here we go,' mutters Young, more to himself than anyone else. He makes the first cut tentatively, just above the navel, a little swooping nick, like a watercolourist gently filling in the foreground on a dreamy, distant landscape. He nicks again, and again, and again, in a perfect vertical line, splitting the skin, no blood yet, gradually making the cut longer until suddenly gravity or weight or tension seems to pull the cut wide. Beneath, a creamy-white moussaka of fat holds off the scalpel for just a couple of cuts, and then he's in, into the guts, probing and pulling. Already his mannequin hands, strangely featureless in their tight white latex gloves, are streaked in bright red blood. The team hand him swabs and clips and forceps. All manner of implements – maybe 60 at a rough count – are laid out, shinily clean, on the steel trolley behind the scrub nurse.

The medical director, searching in the abdomen, starts a running patter for the students, pulling this and that and bits of bowel out of the hole, identifying it, cramming it back. One of the nurses gives a short laugh and asks: 'What next, a white rabbit?'

Everyone grins but no one can see it. In the operating theatre, where all that is visible of the face is the strip between mask and cap, you let your eyes do the laughing. In each glance is a world of expression, in each brow-movement an exaggerated nuance. The medical director stops what he is doing to explain something to the students, and as he does so, bits of innards start emerging of their own volition, pushing up eerily through the hole in the flesh, as if being slowly inflated from below.

It's like cramming too many clothes into too small a suitcase. Open it up and everything pushes out all at once. Or cramming too much into too old a hospital. Let the air in and all kinds of things can pop out.

14

The doctor is angry. He is still young, in his forties, but is already running his own department. He has just come out of a finance meeting and cannot believe he is being asked to justify the same figures, month after month, that he thought had been agreed over a year ago. He has told the management what his patients need, he has shown what the government requirements are, he has benchmarked his service against those provided by other hospitals round the country; he has, he thinks, proved his point. But there is always another meeting, always another wall you run into. That's hospital life. His department is one of the biggest and most prestigious on the site but he feels hamstrung, unable to get anything done. He sits in his shirtsleeves and twirls a biro between his fingers. Through the window behind him, impassive in the sunlight, Parliament lies stretched out along the river, barely listening.

'The first question the finance director asked me was "How do I know you need more beds?" So I benchmarked it, I bloody well got him the data months ago, and at lunchtime today I'm still having to argue the point.'

Why? He shrugs. 'It has just been paralysis here, four years' worth of paralysis since the merger was announced. There's been a lot of work done, but the number of option appraisals I have written out, the number of calculations for this and that, the number of times I have had to re-estimate the number of beds I need . . . you know, when I started off the conversation today I had files of the stuff this thick!' He holds his hands a foot apart.

'I know I need more beds to run a decent service. I know I need more equipment. I know I need a decent out-patients area. I know I need more medical staff. It's no good saying we should move out of London and do it somewhere cheaper, because the patients live *here*. South-east London has a very large resident population of needy people who are deprived and need good care. It's no good if you're not on a major rail link. Guy's and St Thomas' are very well placed. What they need are the money and political will to get it all done. Political will from everyone.'

He sighs and polishes his glasses on his tie. Then he looks uneasy, as if he has spoken out of turn.

15

Try to understand what running a big hospital must be like. Everyone is fighting for a bigger slice of the cake. No one wants to compromise. Everything is a matter of life and death, literally.

Then imagine running and merging two big old teaching hospitals in central London. It is like trying to turn off the waste disposal by sticking your hand down the sink. No one feels too sorry for you when things get messy because they can't see why you did it in the first place.

For the chief executive, the opportunities to shove hands down sinks are endless. At Guy's, Matthews has inherited a huge building project for what is virtually a brand-new hospital, which has already hit long delays and large cost overruns. It has been partially bankrolled by a carpet millionaire with close links to Guy's, who was happy to make a modest donation – modest by comparison with the total cost of construction – and honoured that the building was to be named after him. Once the merger of the two hospitals and the subsequent shift in acute services was announced, the carpet millionaire was not so happy, because his building has been redesignated for planned operations and psychiatric care. He was hoping for something more along the lines of a world-class cancer research centre. He has become a very unhappy carpet millionaire, and something of a public-relations disaster for the new Trust.

Then there is morale. In terms of jobs, the Trust is leaking like a sieve. Like many London hospitals, St Thomas' and Guy's cannot hold on to to low-grade nurses because of low pay and terrible accommodation. The Trust is unpopular with junior doctors because of the hours, the facilities, the academic bureaucracy and what they see as the crusty intransigence of the senior consultants. And it is loathed by many of the older Guy's doctors who have spent five years organising facilities for their new hospital wing only to be told: sorry, we are going to use it for something else. They are furious, and become active participants in a vocal campaign to Save Guy's which draws considerable support from the Kent commuter suburbs. On top of that, everyone on the two sites, from senior doctors down to the youngest of managers, is at each other's throats because they think that merger means rationalisation. Which department will go where? Who will get which space? Who reports to who? What will survive? These issues are difficult enough in a normal hospital without trying to squeeze a rival in on the act too.

And of course hospitals like St Thomas' and Guy's are anything but normal anyway. They are teaching hospitals, which means that they are also part of the academic system, run partially like a university. They get money not just from the local health authorities, to buy care for patients, but also from the Government, to train new generations of doctors, dentists, nurses and technical staff. For a manager, this can have huge benefits – if one source of cash dries up you can squeeze the other; if they have different financial years, you can transfer all kinds of obligations – but it also makes the chain of command rather idiosyncratic. While many of Matthews' clinical staff have NHS contracts with the Trust, others have contracts with the medical school and hence are loyal to a completely different authority. To confuse matters further, under a longstanding custom at St Thomas', some of the staff on NHS contracts also teach and research, and some of the staff on university contracts spend most of their time treating patients. And when you look for the NHS doctors, they seem to be down Harley Street rather a lot, and when you look for the university doctors, they appear (OK, just occasionally) to be in Hawaii or Sri Lanka, where they are lecturing at implausible-sounding conferences. If you were an outside management consultant, you would ask: what is going on? But if you are chief executive, and your senior doctors tell you not to rock the boat, the system has worked for years, don't mess it up, then you probably listen. And you probably follow their advice. It doesn't help you manage, though.

Anyway, you clear the decks and you prioritise. The merger looks like an administrative nightmare to outsiders, but to the chief executive it has a certain logic. Neither hospital could go on as it was; better-sized departments will mean a better range of services, better economies of scale, better teaching and research and, hopefully, better quality of care. That is the theory, anyway. The real difficulty is keeping a normal service going for the community while everything is being changed and 1,000 undergraduates are being taught. It may not be the bit of the Trust's remit that is uppermost in the minds of most of its staff – the Special Trustees paid for the large inscription Serving the Community 24 Hours a Day to be added to the sign on Gassiot House, perhaps as a reminder – but it is the part that gets the worst headlines when anything goes wrong. And it is headlines that bring politicians over the river, sticking their oar in, faster than you can say free publicity.

So you keep calm, you try to avoid cock-ups, and you make sure that the hospital keeps pushing out a trickle of positive stories – that is what the public-relations department is for, after all – to counteract anything nasty that might loom up, like dead bodies behind the pipes, or in the lift, or anywhere else, for that matter. People die all the time in hospitals, but the public and their politicians do not like reading about it, whether human error was involved or not. And most of all, if you are chief executive, you try to get the figures right: money in, money out, number of doctors, number of managers, the right pay, everybody happy. There are all sorts of sleights of hand that can be used. Does around 1,200 managers sound too many for the Department of Health? Easy. Some can keep the same job titles but just change their classification so they are now something else. Everyone does it.

Most of the time, though, Matthews worries about money. Every year he oversees laborious negotiations with some of his main sources of income in the newly created internal market: the health authorities who buy fixed amounts of certain services, and the GP fundholders who are allowed to buy their own care, as and when they want it. But it's not even as easy as that. Despite attempts by successive Conservative governments to introduce real market conditions, everything is skewed by the imperatives. Over two-thirds of medical work and half of surgical work is non-discretionary. In other words, it just turns up in A&E and out-patients unannounced. Other work looks discretionary, but isn't. If you are a major cancer care centre for the south-east, you cannot turn away referrals in the same way as you can someone wanting a hip replacement operation. This gives you a pretty weak negotiating position, as you can never say, 'Sorry, you are not offering enough cash, we are not going to do it.' You have to say, 'We will do this at cost. Please pay us. Please?'

First, of course, you have to work out how to price cost. Actually, it's impossible (few in a real market price at cost, as there are usually too many shared overheads). Instead, you lick your finger and stick it in the air, or read the time off the clock and turn it into pounds and pence. You make assumptions at the start of the year: there will be this many patients going through A&E, there will be such-and-such operations. The purchasers agree to pay an amount; you whittle it away as the work goes through. Then when the lump sum is used up, you close beds and wait for the next financial year, and in the case of operations, bump all your GP fundholders up the list.

Each time, because more patients want more care, and more technology makes more care more expensive, your belt gets tighter. Each time the purchasers ask you to absorb the increases in work with greater efficiency. Each time you argue back that there are real costs involved in taking on the extra work. And at the heart of it all is an unsolvable riddle: how much is a human life worth? What should you spend to save one? Do you have an upper limit? No one knows. Anyway, you argue so long and so hard that by the time you have finished negotiations on one financial round, you have to start negotiations on the next. It is the fiscal equivalent of painting the Forth Bridge. Only the bridge gets longer every time.

And that's before you have even thought about dealing with the doctors, the nurses, the auxiliary staff and everyone else who works, at least nominally, for you. Many of them, you will be surprised to find, you have absolutely no power over whatsoever. Some of them, especially the doctors, seem to live so far in the past that communication is virtually impossible without a time machine. And yet it is hard not to feel sympathy for their predicament. They have witnessed a pace of change virtually unparalleled in any other profession: new technology, new methods of funding, new ways of working. Everything which the older consultants have become accustomed to – the grateful acquiesence of patients, the unquestioning deference of managers, the loyal respect of their own juniors – has been slowly eroded. No one calls them 'sir' any more, few refer to them as Doctor or Mister, everyone is known by Christian names, the mood is one of matey touchy-feeliness. No wonder they ask: how can patients have faith in their diagnoses if there is no distance? How can students trust what they learn if there is no hierarchy? How can junior doctors ever instil confidence if they don't wear a tie?

Matthews knows that, like veteran Rotary Club businessmen left stranded by new ways of management, some of the older doctors feel utterly bemused by hospital medicine in the nineties. They stick their thumbs in their waistcoats, suck on the end of their half-moon glasses and wonder why no one else can see that the place is going to the dogs. You have to live with that. You try and winkle some like-minded people into key positions and see if you can all gingerly guide the vessel by consensus. Sometimes it works.

16

Tony Young smiles curtly at the interruption, a little dig from the hospital's strategy director – 'Have you been taking management classes or something?' – to remind him who does what round here. As medical director, he is the only doctor at the morning's meeting of the Trust Executive. Most of the rest (the strategy director, the finance director, the projects director, the chief executive and the assistant chief executive) are 'suits'. Not he, though. Ever the senior surgeon, he has put on his white coat before entering (despite the fact that he isn't seeing patients for at least an hour), conscious that it is a potent symbol of stature at such a gathering. Only he has confronted death day after day, and held warm life in his latexed hands – a fact they can never ignore. The only other member of the clinical staff on the Executive that morning is the nursing director, a formidable Scotswoman in ruffled blouse and skirt who looks as if she has MATRON stamped right through her like a piece of Edinburgh rock.

'If I may continue?' Young, steel-rimmed spectacles pushed low on his nose, offers a prowling, imperious glance at his colleagues. They sit around a long table eying a plate of biscuits in the middle. A trolley of coffee waits under the projector screen at the other end of the room. A large medical metal sink stands in one corner. Like so many NHS rooms, this one, nestling on the ground floor of the nurses' block, appears to be in its third or fourth reincarnation. Clinical, educational, and now bureaucratic. This is the weekly meeting of the executive directors, the decision-making body that doesn't exist on any of the literature about who runs what at the hospital. Somehow the meetings, known informally as 'Monday morning prayers', have become more important than all the other bodies, committees and gatherings that punctuate and embellish hospital life. Some are just for doctors, some are just for managers, some are for the great and the good and any visiting dignitary who might be soft for a financial squeeze or a publicity opportunity. But here, in this meeting, with the chief executive at the head of the table and the senior suits all around, things really do look as if they are getting decided, or at least considered (the real fear for those in positions of power is that decisions always get taken in the meetings you aren't at). Swift, incisive action is probably not this particular chief executive's style. But that, concludes the medical director, is probably a good thing, given the sensitive nature of the hospital's merger with Guy's. Consensus is what is needed, and consensus is what the doctors and nurses and ancillary staff and patients get. Even if Young, a man used to making up his mind fast – he is, after all, a top surgeon – finds it infuriating at the best of times.

But this morning, a sunny morning, he is in a good mood. His early routine has gone smoothly: up at six at his big house in Blackheath, breakfast with his wife – one Weetabix, one slice of toast, pot of strong Colombian coffee – get dressed, stroll to the station, catch the 7.44 to Waterloo, brisk walk down the York Road, exercising those coronary muscles all the way. A bit of paperwork and then into the meeting. If that makes him sound methodical, then undoubtedly he is, that being one of the key characteristics of his profession. But he is not an earnest man, quite the reverse; in fact he is rather too sharp for a lot of his colleagues' liking. At 52, still handsome, with his fine-featured face, thinning curls and humorous eyes, he speaks well and has the knack of commanding a meeting, no doubt gleaned from many years of teaching and running doctors' committees. And there is more to him than that. He studied fine arts as well as medicine, and lets it be known that he thinks the best doctors are not cerebral intellectuals but Renaissance Men with a facility for communication. He is a moderniser. For him, too many doctors are conservative duffers, a view which sometimes complicates his task of mollifying the opposing factions whose animosity consumes the two hospitals. Suffice to say that some of his peers in the consultants' dining room at St Thomas' think that, like the chief executive, he too is an ambitious man, who rather deserves to be pegged down and have his liver pecked out each week in the endless bureaucracy of hospital-running. That's internal politics for you.

Yet as medical director Young speaks for all doctors, and represents their interests to the executives who run the Trust's business side. As a breast and endocrine specialist of some experience, he also has their respect (though less than many might think, as doctors are generally only interested in their own field). But he has something, a presence or gravitas denied to others. People who meet him side by side with the chief executive often wonder who is the real boss, misunderstanding the true dynamic of hospitals (chaos organised by committee). Running two hospitals at the same time as you are merging various specialisms on to different sites probably requires that something. The problem is there is not a lot of it around.

And being medical director is very much a part-time job. He still has his surgical list to see to: lumps and bumps and varicose veins, and even humble hernias. He also has his occasional private practice (operations at the Churchill) and the conference circuit to attend to. In the past he shared the medical director's post with a professor from Guy's, but the professor stood down, and now he has it to himself. Not for much longer, though: just a few months before a new man takes over and he can really concentrate again on his operating lists. In his world, you cannot step away from the operating table for long; there is always someone younger and sharper waiting to slip into your theatre greens. The medical director's salary of somewhere close to £100,000, before private practice, is compensation, however.

Perhaps most importantly, though, Young is a St Thomas' man. His father was a biochemist at the hospital, and he vividly remembers sitting in the laboratory as a boy, watching goldfish in a tank and loving the feel of it all, the shiny benches and the retort stands, the bustle of quiet industry. He went to Epsom College, one of St Thomas' feeder schools, and got a scholarship to the hospital even before he went to Cambridge. He has spent most of his working life at the hospital and knows how much things have changed. Housemen don't open the door of their surgeons' Rolls-Royces any more, for a start. His own son declined to go to Thomas', and has gone to Edinburgh instead, a sure sign that the old *cosa nostra* is being gradually dismantled. Fewer Masons, fewer white, middle-class boys. The hospital is mutating, changing beyond recognition as the outside world pricks its walls and new influences rush in. He has sat behind bare tables at recruitment fairs watching earnest Asian parents push their sons forward. He sat on committees in the bad old days when Lambeth politicians bankrupted the hospital to embarrass Mrs Thatcher. He watched as the Government responded, appointing their businessmen advisers with a brief to introduce 'more competition' into the system. One of Thatcher's plutocrats even waffled to him: 'Any organisation that can't take 30 per cent of its staff out isn't managing itself properly!' Young got so angry that he almost hit him. The businessman was quite taken aback and never mentioned the idea again. Young feels as though he has seen it all, and nothing really ever surprises him any more, especially not the bish-bosh of merging Thomas' with Guy's. A larger Trust mean better doctors and bigger economies of scale, he is sure of that. Ask him if it means better all-round treatment for patients – prompter care, nicer surroundings, a more humane atmosphere rather than the morale-sapping ambience of a huge illness factory – and he is less convincing.

But right now he is in his element, running through medical matters for the Executive's attention. He leaves the best till last. 'The person in charge of frozen sperm is worried that he is about to commit an offence. Apparently,' he drags out the last syllable for effect, 'we have got gallons of the stuff.'

The suits laugh, a trifle nervously. Frozen sperm is just the kind of thing you can slip up on when you least expect it.

17

A prank on a medical school rugby tour goes too far. A UMDS student produces a syringe in a bar in Plymouth, extracts his own blood, mixes it with vodka and gets another to drink it. There are also allegations of vandalism and sexual assault on the tour. The *Sun* gets hold of the story, describing the students as 'vampires' and louts. A few doctors demand that the offenders are thrown out, but the medical school takes a more lenient view. After all, student high spirits have a certain tradition here. Yet surely, argues one angry physician at a consultants' meeting shortly after, if these were working-class boys on an estate in Lambeth, they would not just be condemned, but probably arrested and locked up as well. Yet because they are nice, middle-class medical students they are allowed to get away with it. What kind of message are we sending out?

The hospital managers are bemused. UMDS, the medical school linked to Guy's and St Thomas' and soon to be joined to King's, appears to be a law unto itself. At times like this the managers feel a mile apart from the medical fraternity, so far away that they couldn't even send them a semaphore signal and guarantee they would see it. The doctors at old hospitals like to do things just so.

18

'I'll tell you what,' says Siobhan. She picks up the coffee pot from the sink in the corner and refills her mug. She has worked at the hospital on and off for over twenty years, first as a practitioner and now as a manager. She is driven and idealistic, but speaks with the bruised resignation of a professional who has spent too many years banging her head against the same brick wall. 'I really don't know if there is still a strong Masonic lodge here, but there is certainly a very Masonic way of doing things. It's very much a boys' network, very much who you know rather than what you can do, and I am speaking as one whose dad is a Mason.

But I think that will get broken down by the influx of female doctors.'

No, the problem, she goes on, is that the attitudes of older doctors are deeply entrenched, and that's all embedded in the rich heritage of an old hospital like St Thomas'. These doctors feel threatened by change, and are extremely uncomfortable with the hospital's position serving a community which is one of the most socially deprived and ethnically diverse in London. So they huddle together for support. St Thomas' is, she says, the only hospital she has ever worked in in which the doctors have a separate consultants' dining room.

'What does that say? It is all about having a culture of not mixing with people who you do not think are at your level socially or intellectually. It holds us all back in terms of development. Let's be frank: St Thomas' has a great reputation but it is no longer at the forefront in terms of innovation and change, and the dining room is symptomatic of that. Saying the merger has held everything back is just an excuse. I worked in a unit where five hospitals were merged together and they didn't have the problems we are having here. But they also did not have the approach that the consultants have here. You can say there's been total paralysis because of the mishandling of the merger, but what people are tending to ignore is that there were big questions being asked even before the merger about what was happening at the hospital in terms of quality of care, evidence-based practice and moving things forward. Did we have a better record at providing NHS care than other London hospitals?' She pauses while she considers her own question. 'Show me the evidence,' she says.

19

Five staff wait for the medical director in a ward up on the tenth floor. The ward is divided into bays around a dog-leg. Four beds, six beds, isolation rooms, shared bath and toilet facilities, a central station for nurses, a television in each bay, wide windows looking out over the Thames and Parliament. If you were well, you could really enjoy the views. But if you were well, you wouldn't be there.

Young wears his white coat over a stripy shirt, monochrome tie and grey pinstripe suit trousers. His name and title are carried in capital letters on a little name badge on his chest. He pushes through the swing doors adjacent to the lifts and gathers up his group by the central station: two white-coated male registrars in their early thirties, a nurse practitioner in dark blue, a ward sister, and an older doctor in shirtsleeves and tie, holding a batch of cards tied together with a loop of string. By this thread hang the patients brought in for operations this afternoon. Now everyone is together, they can be inspected.

Young looks his shirtsleeved junior straight in the eye. 'I think patients prefer to see a white coat,' he says firmly but politely. 'I can see that you have got your name tag so it's not a problem, but I think a white coat is preferable.'

The younger doctor, tall, dark and broad, with jet-black hair pushed back, smiles with a slightly quizzical look, as if he is not sure whether this is a bollocking or not. Young is well liked by his junior staff – he gives them space, lets them laugh and is not a misogynist, unlike some senior surgeons – but he can be a tough taskmaster. The younger doctor nods and attempts to look earnest, while Young gestures at his cards.

'Who's first?'

'Hernia.'

The group follow the doctor to a bay on the left. In a bed under the window lies an elderly man, pink and cherubic and with a grin on his face as wide as the river outside. He is clearly delighted at the attention, and cannot believe his luck at having no fewer than six staff around his bed.

'Would you mind just unbuttoning your pyjama jacket and showing us the hernia, Mr Jones?'

'No, no, of course,' says the man, fumbling his buttons open, taking off the pyjama top and lying back. The group incline their heads as one to study his abdomen. It looks pale and vulnerable in the morning sun. There, to the right of his navel, lies a small wobbly flesh-sac, the size of a baby's fist, pink and wrinkly, like a second scrotum.

Young sits beside him on the bed, quizzing him gently, as if he is just visiting a friend.

'Been in before?'

'Just for my waterworks, Doctor.'

'Oh, yes, I see,' says Young, studying the man's notes. 'Do you mind if we just have a feel?'

He presses round the hernia gently. The junior doctors follow suit – they will be helping him in the operation later – while the nurses watch.

'I'm afraid you'll probably lose your navel, Mr Jones. Can you live with that?'

'Oh, yes,' says the man. He rubs his bare feet together as if in anticipation. The toenails are gnarled and yellow, like rough pebbles. In hospital, everyone seems to have bad toenails. Nothing shows your age more.

The group move to the next-door ward and another bay. The ritual continues. A West Indian woman in a short gown waits to show her varicose veins. Young introduces himself quietly. His manner is soft and polite. He asks: would she mind? He kneels before her like a courtier and runs one hand up and down her dark calf, feeling for the veins. They are hard to see. As he picks them out he draws wiggly lines round them with a dark felt pen. The woman, middle-aged and nervous, looks bemused. Young talks to one of the junior doctors: 'I think we will strip that down to there . . . then that . . . actually, it might be bigger . . .'

He looks up at the patient. 'Can I put my hand on your groin?' he asks, ever so politely. The woman nods. His hand gently rises up her leg. 'OK, now give me a big cough . . .' The woman coughs quietly. 'Fruitier than that if you can.' She coughs more loudly.

'Right,' he says, turning to the other doctors, 'you'll have to take it up to there.'

The woman, who has barely spoken up to now, asks when she will be allowed home after the operation.

'You should be ready to go tomorrow,' he says. Most patients cannot wait to get out, and nowadays, the hospital cannot push them out fast enough. Only the very sick remain.

Two down, two to go. The group moves to another bay. The next patient, a nervous woman in her 50s, is unwilling to expose her hernia for the group. Young says of course, quite understandable, and he helps the ward sister draw curtains round the bed before stepping inside. The other doctors have to wait outside. One rolls his eyes at another. 'It's ridiculous,' he says, 'I'm probably the one doing the operation and she won't let me look at it!' The others laugh. Twenty years ago they would all have inspected the hernia, whatever the patient's misgivings. Now they respect her wishes. That much has changed. Patients' expectations are higher and their power is greater. It rubs up against medical efficacy like a bad case of tennis elbow, but most staff respect it.

Finally, in a small room looking out over Big Ben, the last patient is waiting: a middle-aged man, wearing pants and a pyjama top, with a hernia in the groin. He chats animatedly: his history, who he saw first, when he saw them. Young's tone is blokey but kind. When he asks the man to drop his baggy white pants he does so happily, with hardly a shrug of embarrassment.

He stands there, his bare bum to the Houses of Parliament, his cock retreating shyly into large testicles, looking for all the world as if he is just taking the air. The group study his groin. In fact, most of them can't see anything *but* his testicles.

'Thank you, Mr Smith,' says the medical director as the man pulls up his pants.

Downstairs in the Central Hall, near where the honour boards hang and the portraits of old doctors stare gloomily down from the walls, the main fire alarm is going off. No one takes any notice. It happens every day. The alarm, which is connected directly to the fire station, is faulty. Two or three engines rush up to the back of East Wing most mornings. And most mornings they go home disappointed. Everything carries on regardless. In the corner, equally oblivious to the bell ringing, a pianist pounds away at a grand piano, a little light cultural relief paid for by the Trustees or the Friends or some other well-meaning organisation. Right now, as the medical director crosses the hall in search of his morning bunch of students, it simply seems like a scene from the madhouse.

20

A young doctor, in his twenties, just qualified, articulate, self-assured, is telling a friend how it all works in the medical school: which student gets to go to which jobs, what is decided and by whom. The system at St Thomas', once one of the great bastions of medical patronage, has been tidied up over the years and is now fairly objective, but it has its quirks. He explains:

'So there are around 200 students in my year, all about to qualify, all jostling to see what they can get. The doctors do a roll, listing all the students in the year and ranking them from one to 200. The rankings are based on your exam results and on marks given to you in your firm from your consultant, which is a complete farce as some habitually give great marks and some give crap marks. And then, at the end of this, they have this sort of secret meeting of all the top doctors, and allocate everyone random marks for, well, being captain of the rugby team, having famous relatives ...'

'Oh, come on, that can't be true.'

'Well, OK, it's supposed to be for winning prizes or having special responsibilities, but that's not what we think. Anyway, the point is they are *really* careful about the marks all the way through and then they totally negate it by adding these different marks for different things at the end. We don't really know what they are for, but if you play golf with the right consultants it seems like you do better. That's just how it's perceived. It's totally subjective. So then you end up with a number, a ranking if you like, and the first 100, who are, like, really academic, well connected and probably hopeless at dealing with patients, get campus house-officer jobs at Thomas' and Guy's and the rest get shoved out to other hospitals. You just apply to other places that have links with us, and the same jobs come up every year.'

'Where?'

'Oh, places like Sidcup. You get much better experience there, it's less pressurised and more varied than working here. Here, you just end up doing clerical stuff, filling in forms and fetching X-rays. And the great thing about the jobs outside is that for most of them, you don't have to do any interviews for the posts, you just get them. That's really quite nice.'

'Really?'

'Yeah, it's always been like that. You just say, I'm from Guy's and St Thomas'. Trust me.' And he laughs with the full irreverence of youth.

21

The training manager takes the last flight of concrete steps briskly. 'Follow me, careful how you go,' she shouts to the eighty or so inductees trudging up behind. As part of their induction day tour she likes to take them up to the top of North Wing on to the roof, to see the view over London. To access the roof, she borrows a key from Facilities which lets her through the machinery room at the top of the block.

'This way,' she says, turning the final corner. 'Oh . . .'

Sitting at the top of the stairs is a heavily pregnant woman, sharing a large joint with her Rastafarian boyfriend. Their jaws drop at the sight of the group now blocking the stairway beneath them. A sly titter ripples through the inductees.

'Excuse *me*,' says the training manager, reaching for her key.

22

It's two in the morning when Jim decides he's had enough. An eerie calm has settled on A&E. One old man sits in the main waiting room watching television. At the reception the triage nurse – everyone gets assessed as they walk in, it makes sense and it's good for the statistics – reads a book. The receptionist sits silently at her side. You can barely hear the traffic now, just the occasional chug of a late-night taxi outside.

Jim goes to talk to the sister in Major Treatment, just mopping up the last of the post-pub entries. The drunks. The collapses. A pair of cheery green-uniformed ambulancemen push an empty trolley-bed past. A faint smell of faeces hangs in the air. A good-looking nurse with a mop and bucket, wearing small white galoshes, squeaks past. 'Yes, I know,' she smiles at Jim, 'I'm looking pretty attractive tonight!' Jim tries to concentrate on the matter in hand.

'I'm going now,' he says, scanning the sister's face for any sign of irritation. She's OK this one, he gets on with her. You have to get on with them: the sisters are the linchpins of the department, the bearings on which the whole hospital mechanism runs, but they are all different. Some give you a smooth ride, others don't. Jim is still in trouble with one for not pulling aside a junior doctor who dared to criticise a nurse in a report. That kind of thing – taking sides, closing ranks – gets people's necks bristling. Jim always aims for a smooth ride, a laugh and a joke, be serious when you need to be.

Sex complicates it, as he's never quite sure who is dating who. It's a simple fact that the younger doctors and nurses are at it constantly – it's the stress, of course – and hospitals are the last place in the world you can keep a secret. Everyone wants to know who snogged who at the last party. It's always been a bit like that. The difference now is that it's the nurses always joking about the lack of George Clooney lookalikes, rather than the other way round. The women doctors guard their tongues. Some feel they get a much rougher ride from female nurses than from any of the hospital's men.

Jim tells the sister to phone if anything urgent comes in and waves goodbye. He goes round the back and throws his white jacket across the chair in the little office he shares with the other registrars, then wanders back out through the reception. The electronic doors slide open. Outside, the stars are bright even above the urban glare. Jim wanders down the concrete ambulance ramp to where he has parked his battered old car, illegally, in a little alcove on the way up. He needs to get home. He has to be up early to do a shift in Intensive Care. He breathes in and out slowly, loudly, mimicking the distinctive sound of a ventilator machine, usually the only noise audible in the anxious stillness of an Intensive Care ward. He chuckles. The tawdry bulk of the hospital rises up behind him, grimy, still and tense. In just a few hours it will open up properly again, full of life and death and bustle and a whole new day. *Bring me your poor, your . . .*

Intensive Care. He frowns. Like watching paint dry, he murmurs to himself, and drives wearily home.

THOSE LITTLE SCREWS
OF EXISTENCE

I would suggest that one of the fundamental reasons why so many doctors become cynical and disillusioned is precisely because, when the abstract idealism has worn thin, they are uncertain about the value of the actual lives of the patients they are treating. This is not because they are callous or personally inhuman: it is because they live in and accept a society which is incapable of knowing what a human life is worth.

John Berger, *A Fortunate Man*

If Florence Nightingale were carrying her lamp through the corridors of the NHS today, she would almost certainly be searching for the people in charge.

Sir Roy Griffiths, report on NHS management, 1983

1

It's the sound that catches you first. The faint hum and blip of the metal boxes, the phtt-pok of the ventilator, the distant squelch of an anaesthetist's theatre boots on his way through from surgery. Yet nobody speaks. It's as hushed as a church. The relatives sit. The nurses wait. The doctors write notes. The patients lie unconscious. Sometimes it's so quiet you could hear a needle pop skin. Only the machines break sweat, driving fluids into the bodies, pumping the medications through, forcing the lungs to breathe, getting the balance of gases right. In Intensive Care, technology takes over. In Intensive Care, modern medicine reaches its apotheosis.

But Intensive Care is also one-on-one, patient and nurse. Without someone being able to read the machines, analyse the results and understand the patient's physiology, the technology is worse than useless. It is dangerous. Good Intensive Care nurses take a lot of training. They have to deal with maths and mechanics and physiology in a constantly changing world. They have to have a different kind of mind from most nurses. They end up knowing easily as much as a senior house officer. Then they see the young doctors looking at them with big eyes when a patient is going off, pleading: what do I do now, help me, please? An experienced nurse will say: it's OK, do such-and-such, take this test, look at this, if it's this we will do this, and they say: right, fine. They breathe a sigh of relief. Thank God the nurse knows. But good Intensive Care nurses are expensive and always in short supply. From that supply problem a stack of consequences flips over like a line of cards. No nurses, no beds. No beds, no operations. No operations, no patients. Long waiting lists. The surgeons are left sitting around playing bridge on full salary while GPs wonder where else they can send people and trust managers wonder what the hell is going wrong with their figures.

But the job? It takes a certain type of personality. Intensive Care units are notoriously cliquey and more than a little addictive. Those who love it say there is nothing like it. Just one patient who is your sole responsibility. Total patient care. There is the buzz of receiving someone in trauma, unstable, close to death, everything going wrong, and by your efforts and those of your colleagues, a few hours later that patient has a steady blood pressure, their urine is flowing, they are calm, they are sleeping, and you feel you have done something. You can almost touch what you have done. It is tangible.

At other times it is deeply frustrating. You are nursing people who should never have been resuscitated in the first place. You are looking after patients who you know deep in your heart are not going to survive. You are coming into work going: please let everything go all right tonight, please let everything go all right tonight, and then you look at the staff mix balanced against the patient needs and your heart sinks. You are cleaning up the mess that modern medicine sometimes leaves behind.

Cathy knows about Intensive Care. She was an Intensive Care nurse before moving into management. She is vigorous, brown-haired, square-built, attractive in a dependable, cope-in-all-situations type of way. Trained initially in the Midlands and then at St Thomas', she has spent half her life at the hospital and has a devotion to the institution common among such veteran professionals. Now she is a senior manager, with an office in the decrepit-looking block called Riddell House that runs beside Lambeth Palace Road. Riddell House will be pulled down to make way for the next big building project at Thomas', a new women and children's hospital, if the chief executive can get the money from somewhere. Right now it houses anything that can't fit anywhere else: offices, meeting rooms, mice. It's a spillover block.

Cathy has seen nearly all the changes in Intensive Care since it was pioneered forty-odd years ago. The first Intensive Care unit at Thomas' was built in 1966. Now everything is different: the technology has changed, the type of patients have changed, the expectations have changed. There is enormous political pressure on managers to ensure that Intensive Care works smoothly. Without it, so much else at the hospital falls apart.

She talks robustly, with the confidence of someone who has seen governments and policies come and go, but the hospital sur-vive. Yet she knows the sands are shifting again and is obviously perplexed at the arguments over funding, and over how much more should be poured into Intensive Care at the expense of other priorities. Like so many others, she sees all the contradictions, and doesn't know if any answers will ever be found.

'These last few days it has been quite quiet. Intensive Care tends to go in peaks and troughs and you never know why. But down periods are not occurring with anywhere near the frequency they used to. In the old days we took patients from anywhere but now they have to have a contract. That bit worries me; the business manager has to chase all that sort of thing up. What they wanted to do was flatten out the hierarchy, and all they have done is create another hierarchy not filled with nurses but with people with pound signs for eyeballs. A lot of people feel angry about it . . .

'Equally I understand that there are areas in the country that don't get the same service as central London. That poor boy who had to travel 55 miles to get an Intensive Care bed, that was criminal. But I also know that if you cram people into Intensive Care without the right number of staff there will be an accident, something will happen due to neglect or someone not being there, an alarm will go off or a machine fail and that person will end up in a coroner's court and it wasn't their fault. How do you cope with that?

'Deep down, though, I know that nursing standards are not as good, and lots of nurses will agree. They are there by the skin of their teeth doing the best that they can. They rarely go home saying, "Yeah, that was a good day." They go home worrying, "Oh, I didn't do this," or "I didn't talk to him."

'But the thing is, people expect more nowadays. That man up north who died in transit with the cerebral bleed: I heard on the network that he had such a catastrophic bleed that nothing could be done for him but they carried on, for whatever reasons or whatever pressures. Often it is the relatives and the power of the media. They say, "I will go to the papers if you don't do it!" You don't think about it on a day-to-day basis, but you do as you go higher up the scale. All the time you have to think: what would the press make of this?'

2

Matt Tee is 34, two years in the job as head of public relations for the Trust. He looks young – medium height, broad face, sharp smile, Mandelson hair cut – but he is well connected and knows about oiling the right wheels. He is New Labour classless, Arsenal season-ticket holder, born to well-off parents in this patch of south London, educated at Johanna Primary in Lower Marsh by the Old Vic Theatre, and Pimlico Comprehensive, where Jack Straw used to be chair of governors. Like many who have ended up as Labour Party workers, he started as a student union rep before working round the public sector, first as a teacher then as a trainer. In the early nineties he coached prospective MPs in campaign skills, and later joined Neil Kinnock's tour team for the ill-fated 1992 general election. Tee's job was to check out the venues for Kinnock's pre-election visits. He would go in the day before, confirm the hotel bookings, sort out where to put the barriers for the factory visit, where to park the drop-off coaches, how to do the tour round the marketplace so Kinnock didn't get photographed under the Nutty Fruit Bar sign. All that sort of stuff. He was there with Kinnock in Wales on election night when the results came in. He was there when Kinnock kicked the wall and shouted: 'What the fuck have I spent the last nine years doing?'

Tee moved into PR after the election because it was the best offer he got. The work started in dribs and drabs, a bit for a health authority, some research for a council, advice for a charity. There were plenty of left-leaning public-sector bodies who couldn't pay proper PR fees but needed some media nous, especially as Conservative government reforms were bringing packs of reporters panting on to their doorstep. Tee described his clients as the 'not-for-profit' sector – the joke being that they didn't pay enough to be for his profit either. Not to worry. His wife worked, lecturing in training, and he had enough money to get a mortgage on a five-bedroom repossession in Herne Hill. He was OK. But he liked the people. He had a knack, engrained from his background, for getting on with everyone, posh and poor alike. A few months' work quickly stretched into three years. Then he saw the job of head of public relations at the Guy's & St Thomas' Trust advertised in the *Guardian* and decided he needed a change. He applied for it and eight interviews later, he was in.

It was not that surprising, really. This was his neighbourhood, he could put names to faces, he had even been chair of the Bermondsey Labour Party for a bit. That local knowledge was invaluable: a trust has to watch the local politicians as keenly as the national ones. The Labour link was a worry, according to his first interviewing panel, though by then, halfway through John Major's final term, perhaps the Trust could feel which way the wind was turning.

It's a big job: six staff, budget close to £250,000, a brief that stretches from handling relations with Parliament to fixing up footballers for children's ward visits at Christmas. Tee learnt a lot quickly (first up: you don't call it PR in a hospital, as any nurse will tell you that PR means 'per rectum' . . .). Much of his job is simply acting as gatekeeper to the media, letting them in, showing them round, introducing them to the right people. The hospital, under the last public-relations chief, had a policy of keeping people out – so much so that health writers complained that doctors at the Trust were gagged. Tee reversed that. Everyone is welcome, unless there is a very good reason to shut the door in their faces.

So he deals with requests for briefings from broadsheet journalists, requests to shoot reports on the wards from news crews, requests to interview doctors for documentaries, requests to help writers researching new drama series. It never stops. Media interest in health has climbed faster than the number of patients in A&E. There is the internal communication to supervise too: posters, the monthly staff newspaper, special announcements. He walks around a lot, introduces himself to heads of department, constantly tries to get a feel of what is going on at both sites. He wants to be the first to know if anything goes wrong. He wants to be the chief executive's eyes and ears. He is tight with Matthews – everyone knows that.

The doctors kept their distance at first. His predecessor had been famously fierce – sometimes he felt she was still there, an unseen presence at every meeting he took in his first few months. But gradually the doctors softened. Most realised how useful public relations could be in a world of competing trusts and internal markets. A few, of course, were rather alarmed at Tee's techniques: sitting on stories till they could be used to snatch publicity from rivals, or whipping up headlines for some gosh-golly research. They just thought any amount of money spent on that sort of thing when the hospital was starved of cash for new equipment was simply another sign of how ridiculous everything had got.

But Tee has never had any doubts that his department is worth the money. There is not just more media interest in hospitals; there are, as he puts it, simply more audiences that need 'looking after', not least the Trust's own staff. But the real reason why he loves and values his job is the belief he has that, despite the fact that the hospital always needs more money, and despite the fact that it doesn't treat patients as quickly as it would like to, it still provides a damn good service. Some might want to portray the situation as the reverse: that the hospital is failing, that the hospital is in crisis. It isn't. He passionately believes that if you come in as a patient, you will receive the best-quality medical care you can get, and he doesn't want people's faith undermined. One day, he admits, things might reach the stage where he thinks people's faith *should* be undermined. But it hasn't got there yet.

Of course, after what happened with the last public relations chief, a lot of the doctors and staff are just grateful he is a man.

3

The young manager paces her office while she talks. She says she doesn't know what it is about hospitals, but there is something going on under the surface that you don't get in other workplaces. 'It's the big element of flirtation that goes on in this place. There's definitely an undercurrent, and it's to do with the strong male culture that still exists here. We took the top management team and the senior doctors away for a weekend to the management college at Cranfield, and this management consultant sat next to me at dinner and said he couldn't believe the level of sexual innuendo in this place. He just couldn't believe it. Managers *and* doctors. And it's true. I can remember meetings with male doctors in here and they get far too close. They are not aware of what they are doing half the time. Women don't know quite how to handle it. I have meetings with one doctor and I can see him undressing me. The way he looks at me. He is such a flirt.'

4

The reason why doctors and staff are grateful that Tee is a man is as follows: three years after the Tomlinson enquiry, the chief executive's deft touch for public relations let him down. Right in the middle of the acrimonious negotiations over how Guy's and St Thomas' would merge, when doctor was pitted against doctor, and powerful forces were looking for ways to undermine the new management, his enemies got a useful piece of information. It was given to the *Daily Mirror*. The paper headlined the story CHAMPAGNE CHEAT: CHIEF EXECUTIVE OF GUY'S AND ST THOMAS' HOSPITAL TRUST HAS SECRET LOVE CHILD.

The chief executive, so adept at patiently unravelling other people's problems, had tangled his own life in knots.

Top health chief Tim Matthews has fathered a secret love child, the *Daily Mirror* reveals today. The champagne-loving boss was thought to have ended his affair with blonde PR girl —, 33, who is on his staff, but their baby — was born 11 weeks ago.

Not only had Matthews, married with two sons, conducted a rather indiscreet affair with his own public-relations chief for many months, he had compounded the problem by promising to end the affair, then fathered a child a year later.

Asked about the baby, he looked visibly shaken and said: 'I am not prepared to make any comment.' Flamboyant Mr Matthews, 43, is Britain's best-paid NHS Trust chief.

The newspaper dug out the information from the register of births while the public-relations chief was away on maternity leave. She had never told colleagues who the father was.

A Trust insider said last night: 'The board are not going to be very pleased with Matthews. They may have forgiven him for having an affair with a member of staff, but whether they will forgive him for fathering an illegitimate child is another matter.'

No one is quite sure how Matthews survived. Doctors at St Thomas' heard that their colleagues at Guy's were gleefully petitioning the Department of Health for the chief executive's removal. The Trust board was horrified by the scandal. What timing! But they backed him. So did his wife. So did the senior doctors at St Thomas'. Better the manager you know, they reasoned, than one you don't.

A Trust spokesperson said: 'This is now a matter of history and not one of current consequence.'

From then on everyone just avoided the subject. Certainly no one said anything about it at Tee's job interviews. The whole farrago was airbrushed out of hospital history faster than Trotsky out of Lenin's Russia. It just sank out of sight, like a stone in a pond, with only faint ripples remaining. One of which was a new PR chief,

Tee. Another was a new Trust chairman for the chief executive to report to, an ex-admiral and stickler for discipline who used to run the Trident missile programme. Quite how his specialist interests dovetailed with those of a hospital trust was uncertain, but life must go on.

5

A teaching hospital is a breeding ground for specialisms. In their variety and spread they reproduce like fungi on a test plate, a little whorl here, a big growth there. Antenatal, cardiology, day surgery, dermatology, diabetes, endocrinology, dietetic, ear, nose and throat, eyes, genito-urinary, gynaecology, haemophilia, HIV, hearing, lipid, midwifery, neurology, oral surgery, orthopaedics, physiotherapy, plastic surgery, radiotherapy, rheumatology, thoracic, X-ray. You can attend out-patients' clinics for each of these specialisms at St Thomas'. Then there are the support services like pathology, radiology, nuclear medicine, pharmacy and nutrition. All human life is here. All human death too.

The specialisms are divided into departments, and the departments headed by directors, who are doctors, backed by managers. They run their own empires. Sometimes they operate in complete isolation from what occurs in any other department in the hospital, even the one next door. At other times they are totally intertwined in a string of services overhauling and rebuilding the sick patient as he or she moves efficiently down the production line. It is as purposeful as any digestive tract, but of course it is never that simple. Every patient has his own story. Every patient takes time. Behind every activity, every referral, every small piece of advice, looms the requisite data and paperwork. Even at the end of the 20th century, when information technology has transformed every other part of society, in hospitals it has made perilously slow progress. It requires investment; so does everything else. It gets prioritised, but then so does everything else too. And it gets stolen, so it is only slowly bought.

Soon, if you are a doctor/manager, a morass of meetings surrounds you, and a mountain of paperwork looms overhead. You run round in circles to stop from sinking. You never shove the system, in case a Matterhorn of form-filling topples over and crushes you.

6

'OK, let's see what we've got.'

Dr Nigel Bateman, top lung man, picks up the photocopied list and taps his pen on the name at the top. One of the young doctors opposite looks at him expectantly, waiting for his cue. Bateman nods at him.

'Mr Jarvis came in with acute . . .'

A nervous air of concentration settles over the room as the young doctors take turns to run through yesterday's admissions. Bateman rests the list on the table in front of him and annotates it methodically, pinching his lips together with the thumb and forefinger of his left hand and nodding his head as he listens. He is a slim man, tall, pale-eyed and sandy-haired, in his mid-fifties, firm but brusque in manner, more like a military engineer than a doctor. As the senior physician 'on take' the day before – and hence responsible for all admissions to the hospital between 8 a.m. and 9 p.m. on that day – he has to work out who he is going to see again on his morning ward round. That is the nature of being on take, the second line of defence after the consultants and registrars in A&E. You filter the sickest patients through the system, working out who should go where. Then the next day you try and find them again. Since the last lot of hospital reforms ditched the idea of specific wards for specific doctors, patients under observation or waiting for treatment can end up anywhere. A morning's ward round can then become a three-hour trek around eight different locations.

It is 8.30 in the morning. The group are loosely huddled around a table in one of the staff meeting rooms in A&E. The faces are young because it is the registrars and junior doctors who have born the brunt of the load the day before. The older ones sit in shirtsleeves and smile nervously as they add their comments. The youngest stand with hands deep in the pockets of their white coats, fists balling up against the dark little reference works they carry there. Occasionally one doctor will flash a knowing grin at a colleague, but generally everyone is on best behaviour. No bad jokes, no sick humour. Dr Bateman, as well as being physician on take, is a respected thoracic specialist and while not a cold man, he has a certain relentless precision in his manner that discourages facetiousness.

The talk is swift: they detail yesterday's events and run through patients' potassium, glucose and gases, crash calls to Resus and who can get beds where. In the corner a dapper man with close-clipped grey hair takes notes studiously. He is wearing a sports jacket and tie, with a little red Aids Awareness ribbon clipped to his lapel. He is the bed manager, Bob, an ex-nurse who controls which patient goes where in the hospital. Everyone calls him Bob the Bed. When the doctors have finished, he makes a brief announcement, pointing out that they are closing 12 beds on one ward because of refurbishment work and opening another 10 in a different ward later in the year.

'Is that official news everyone can talk about,' asks Bateman, 'or unofficial news?'

'Official,' says Bob the Bed. His Scottish accent is soft and slightly guttural, as if he is speaking through a mouthful of boiled sweets. He smiles handsomely.

'So there is going to be a lot of confusion for the next few weeks in the hospital,' says Bateman, in a matter-of-fact manner for the benefit of the younger doctors. If there is an edge of cynicism in his comment, it is barely noticeable.

Bateman's ward round starts up in one of the admission wards, where his team await him. The senior registrar is male, fair-haired, with wide shoulders and a knowing smile. The junior registrar is female, tall and thin, with a calm face belied by nervous hands. The senior house officer is noticeably younger, male, well spoken, with the smart, short haircut and eager manner of a trainee banker. They have worked with the consultant for varying periods and have as much confidence as each position allows. They cluster round a large yellow beehive box whose long, thin drawers overflow with patients' notes.

The senior registrar introduces the first patient, a young West Indian woman with shell-shocked eyes who lies on her side, very still, her hands tucked beneath the pillow. The four doctors stand round her bed, in a four-patient bay off the main ward corridor. A sister pulls the curtains round the bed, the first act in the prolonged, theatrical process of drawing and undrawing that underpins the day's work with metronomic regularity. Shut open next. Shut open next. And each slow dusk a drawing-down of blinds.

The conversation behind the curtains is audible to all, interspersed by the patient's whispered replies and wheezy, rasping cough. The doctors gently bombard her with questions and commands. Where is the pain? Do you feel your tummy is very full? Do you normally cough like that? It sounds as though it is not all cough. Open wide, would you please, say ah ... No, it's not really awful. I don't really know why your temperature is where it is. It sounds as if you have some phlegm to cough up. If you could, we would like to look at it.

After each bed visit, the doctors cluster over the beehive again to amend the looseleaf notes, held together by thin string ties. 'I don't think we have got the solution to this lady yet,' says Bateman, honestly. They move to the next on the list. As the three men walk in front, the junior registrar lags behind with the sister. 'I like your new hair,' she says, with a smile. 'Oh, thanks,' says the sister.

They move from bed to bed, ward to ward. Some patients are sicker than others. Can you hear me, Mr Jarvis? Can you move your right hand, Mr Jarvis? Now move your left hand? Squeeze my fingers, good, squeeze the other hand. Thank you, sir, I just want to listen to this side.

Bateman calls all the male patients 'sir', but without obsequiousness or deference. It is more jovial and chivvying, a manner copied by his subordinates. Occasionally the registrar gets to work as chief barker. He shouts into the ear of an elderly patient: 'GOOD MORNING, SIR! DR BATEMAN IS HERE TO SEE YOU NOW!' Only female patients are addressed by their surnames. Perhaps 'madam' would sound too tart.

The junior registrar scribbles twice as many notes as the others. She has to run the patients, ensuring the consultants' instructions are correctly carried out, liaising with the nursing staff and dealing with anything that comes up between times. With patients spread among a host of different wards, it can be an exhausting business, bleeped from one building to the next. The drug lists, especially for patients with respiratory problems, are long and complicated, and the samples, endless little pots of phlegm coughed up by patients who are generally too ill to spit accurately, invariably messy.

As the morning progresses, the slow rhythm of the wards envelops the doctors' progress. The curtains are drawn, patients shuffle by, cleaners push long, wide brooms slowly, orderlies wander through. Occasionally the process is broken by the unexpected. A patient looks startled when the pay-telephone next to his bed suddenly starts to ring. He answers it, holding the receiver as if it was someone else's urine sample. 'Bed 19? I don't know where bed 19 is,' he says, turning to the doctors. 'Do you know where bed 19 is?'

In the bay opposite, an old man seeks consolation from the nurse taking his blood pressure. 'And the doctor said it was a stroke this time. That's not so good, is it? I tell you, I was so frightened ...' Next to him another man, in pyjamas and dressing gown, is making his own bed, smoothing out the top blanket again and again, as if rubbing out the wrinkles will put his own life into order as well.

To the next bed, the next ward, the next set of curtains. When you came in, sir, you were terribly breathless and horribly wheezy. Which bit of you is still wrong? Still got a pain across the front when you cough? *Cough, cough, hoick.* Yes, that is what I was expecting, some really nasty big phlegm. Oh, yes, it is beastly. What you have got is an infection, hence the pain in the cough. We're going to give you lots of different medicines to attack it in different ways. When will you be able to go home? Well, it's early days. The cultures of the urine and phlegm samples you gave us will come through to us at the end of the day. While you are just sitting there I would like to get a look at your back. *Cough, cough, hoick, spit, waaargh!* Oops, we have got to get a bit more accuracy with that. I'll get someone to clear it up.

They visit a man who they admitted the week before. He lies by the window on a Thameside ward. Behind him, beyond the thick, double-glazed glass, London buses pootle silently over Westminster Bridge, looking like Dinky replicas. The man is young, fit-looking, in his late 30s, and racked by a terrible cough. He says his work frequently takes him to south-east Asia. The doctors thought he'd picked up TB. The tests show he hasn't. Bateman feels the man's stomach and then places his stethoscope on his back, listening to his lungs.

'I can't hear crackles on either side,' he says to his team. 'So what we have got is a man with a bad cough and a chest X-ray that is not particularly impressive.'

The patient grimaces. 'I really want to get rid of this bloody cough, Doctor. In terms of TB, can I get a vaccination against it?'

Bateman looks slightly surprised. 'For the future? Well, there's no evidence that the TB vaccine works after 40. If vaccinated you could do yourself a lot more harm than if you just behave intelligently. If you think you're immune because you are vaccinated you probably won't report any symptoms because you will think you can't get it. The problem is we just don't have the perfect vaccine.'

They move on. There are asthma sufferers to see, pregnant women with respiratory problems, and patients who the consultant hasn't even met before but about whom other doctors want his opinion. He swoops on each ward with his team fanned out behind him like flying swans, darting for the patient list, nosing out the right initials against each name up on the white board. The wards change: each has its own atmosphere, its own sickness level instantly audible. In the very sick wards you hear barely anything: a spattering of low chat, the occasional beep of a machine, and a low, pervasive, mechanical rumble like air-conditioning or a large fridge. In others the volume of bustle and noise feels like a release.

Bateman, who has seen it all before so many times, maintains his upbeat demeanour throughout. Only the little things unsettle him now. He is genuinely excited when his SHO says he has found a patient with calcified coronary arteries which show up in X-ray. 'Fantastic!' he says. 'Bring it along on Wednesday for my students.' Then, within a minute, he is totally horrified when another patient, after pleading for sleeping pills because his cough kept him awake all night, asks when he can have a cigarette again. Bateman's lips purse. The patient – middle-aged, crop-haired, with distinctive tattoos down each arm – quickly attempts to retrieve the situation.

'But oi've bin smokin' since oi was firteen. Oi used t'drink a bottle'a whisky a day too but oi've given that up . . .'

Trying to cure people who insist on damaging themselves is one of the consultants' continual frustrations. Bateman doesn't answer the man, but simply turns and walks out of the bay, shaking his head and leaving his team grinning from ear to ear. He tries not to think: what a waste of money.

7

On the fourth or fifth interview for the public-relations job, Tee was introduced to the medical director who used to share the job with Young. He asked Tee straight away: 'With the money we are planning to pay you I could almost get a consultant – why shouldn't I?'

'That's a legitimate question,' said Tee, stalling while he composed the right reply. Then he ran through what he had told the others: that the hospital had to work in a more competitive environment and address more audiences than ever before; that good communication was essential for efficiency and morale and a host of other things; that news imperatives dictated that reporters would frequently take matters out of context and look for crisis and collapse and catastrophe, and try and play trust off against trust; and that if the hospital didn't have a strategy for dealing with that, then it would get shafted. If it got shafted it would get fewer patients, less money, less research, and they would all lose their jobs – well, they had lived through the late eighties. They knew how close it had been. And anyway, Tee might have added, much of the money for the PR department didn't come from the Trust anyway. It came from the Special Trustees, and was augmented by whatever the PR department could raise in the way of location fees for filming and suchlike. It wasn't as if it had been pulled from anyone's budget for doctors. In short, it would be stupid *not* to have a PR department. So many of the NHS's problems were linked to communication: not explaining to outsiders what was going on, not telling staff why change was necessary. It was vital to morale, and keeping morale up meant better care for patients. And after all, that was what a hospital was all about, wasn't it?

8

Andy is riding down Kennington Road when it happens. A white Nissan, parked ahead of him, indicates and pulls out hard, intent on a fast U-turn. Andy jams his thumb on the hooter button of his motorbike and sees the car stop dead, blocking his path. Andy is a teacher. He thinks rationally. He has been in accidents before. He's been riding for twelve years. He knows he has two choices. In less than three seconds he is going to hit the side of the car at 40 m.p.h. He could jump, let the bike take the impact and hopefully get away with a few grazes, maybe a broken bone. Or he could try and avoid the car, steer round the bonnet, miss any oncoming traffic, save the bike and maybe come out unscathed. Later, he remembers that it was love that got in the way. He was going to see Caroline the next day, Sunday. It was a long drive. He didn't want to miss her, so he chose option two. Stay on the bike.

Wrong choice.

Warm, wet, sticky blood. Blood on his jeans. The driver trying to get him up under the armpits to move him.

'Don't move me. DON'T MOVE ME!'

He's conscious, that's good. He knows that's good. He feels in control. He can see the tarmac under his visor. He feels the road.

He can see feet, people around him. It's OK, he's conscious, he keeps telling himself that, he's not dead, that's good. He can't see the bike. Electric-blue BMW. He loves that bike. What happened? The bastard who had stopped started again just as he swerved round him. The car smashed straight into him. The driver hadn't seen him. The bike went off sideways underneath him. Andy's tall, gangly body spun over the bonnet. His knee was smashed. He remembers his head hitting the tarmac – it felt like ten tons of steel dropping on his helmet. He must be in the road, he needs to move in case he gets run over. He tries to move. YAAARGH! The pain in his hip is so great he almost passes out. The blow to his knee has smashed his thigh up through his hip socket. Then the guy tries to move him. He stops when Andy screams again.

He thinks: at least I have stayed conscious. Suddenly a police-man is there, then a paramedic and ambulancemen. Andy's mind is working hard, fighting the shock and pain. The paramedic is calm and reassuring. 'Don't move,' he says. 'Don't do anything.' Three of them gently, ever so gently, take his helmet off. Andy sees a witness is talking to the policeman.

'Have you talked to her? I want you to talk to her. She saw it all. I feel very aggrieved about this!' The policeman tries to reassure him. Andy can see his trousers are ripped. The ambulancemen are already cutting his clothes off him. The one-piece waterproof suit. His jeans. They are strapping him to a board and giving him gas, asking him where the pain is. He can see the driver of the Nissan, standing, looking on forlorn.

As Andy is loaded into the ambulance the man comes forward and shakes his leg in a desperate gesture of reassurance. Andy screams and hisses to the ambulancemen: 'Keep that man away from me!'

Andy's thoughts are jumbled by the gas. He gives a start as the doors whoosh open at A&E and he feels the warmth of the reception room roll over him. A strange sense of elation hits him. This is like television! They are talking about me as an RTA. It's OK, it's a drama. I'm a real RTA!

Then it all stops and slows down. He's lying there with a policeman and an ambulanceman beside him. He cannot believe how slowly the nurse is walking over to him. He hears snippets of conversation. What are we going to do with him? We're a bit busy at the moment? They can't be saying that! Then he's trundled off again into Resus. It feels like a cubicle. A surgeon comes in. He looks at him, then disappears. Andy wonders what's going on. He is still on the board. He is really uncomfortable. It feels as if someone has thrust a red-hot spanner in his hip. He tries to suck in as much as he can from the bottle of gas. It's not working. The pain.

'I want more, I want more,' he pleads with a nurse. She talks with a doctor. He agrees that he will give him some morphine. They tell Andy they don't want to move him till he has been X-rayed. A policeman asks him for phone numbers of people to tell. He gives them the number of his girlfriend, and of a friend he is meeting for a drink that night. He doesn't want the policeman to tell his parents. He doesn't want to worry them.

Eventually he gets his morphine. Nothing happens. He gets confused. They X-ray him and take him off the board. Suddenly he feels free, as if he is floating above it. Later, he remembers a doctor showing him the X-rays, and explaining that his leg is out of its socket and they will have to put it back. Of course, he says, of course. Then he is being wheeled into an operating theatre by a porter, and he is telling the porter: 'God, this is a great place, it's real fun, isn't it?' and laughing and joking. The porter looks at him with an amused smile and says he's not like most of the people he wheels out of A&E. 'Why's that?' asks Andy. Oh, most of them are insulting us, effing and blinding, trying to hit us, says the porter. As Andy drifts off before his first operation he thinks: it's odd, maybe this is quite a rough place, after all.

*   *   *

Andy wakes up on a ward, in a four-bed bay. He is wearing a hospital gown. His first thought is: YIPPEE! LESS PAIN! I am going to be walking out of here tomorrow. It feels so much better. What a place!

The next morning the surgeon comes to see him. He is friendly and brusque, very public school, just what Andy expects from a hospital doctor. He says that the operation was a success and they have put the leg back in its socket but there is bad news. The socket is smashed. They need to think what to do next. 'We will have to make some decisions as to what to do with you,' he says, finally. Andy feels as if he has hit the tarmac again, this time without a helmet. Then he feels a wet ripple of fear wash over him like a cold wave. If he can't walk, he is going to be here for a long time. That means using a bedpan for weeks. He cannot face using a bedpan. He has always dreaded this. He keeps thinking: I am not going to get out of here. I am not going to get out of here.

The consultants come and go. Andy feels he is being passed from one to another like pass-the-parcel, each one taking another wrapper off, each one getting closer to the nub of the problem. Eventually a man comes to his bedside and introduces himself as a pelvic specialist. He is in his early fifties, bespectacled, grey-haired, unassuming and cautious, not like other doctors Andy has seen, who appear more cavalier, more rugby club in tone. This one never barks orders to his housemen. He speaks to them quietly and courteously.

He tells Andy that he will operate on him this Friday, but they have to do some tests first, different types of X-rays. A bacon-slice scan. All sorts of things that Andy doesn't quite understand.

When Andy goes for an X-ray, the radiologist tells him that his surgeon is the only man in London who does this kind of operation, using a technique which he learnt in France. He has a special operating table made just for his operations. Andy wonders what it does.

Andy likes his ward. His four-bed bay is high up in the North Wing, warm and sunny. He has a stunning view of Parliament. He can sit there for hours, just looking at the view. It is extraordinary: blue sky, grey river, Parliament newly cleaned and looking as fastidious in its Gothic uprightness as a prisoner's matchstick model. A friend brings him some clothes. He wears an old T-shirt, rather than pyjamas. He feels comfortable.

But the other patients in his bay are a shock. An elderly man on his right has a wasting bone disease, and looks close to death. His head is sunk into his shoulders. Opposite is a West Indian rude boy with heavy attitude. He has had an operation to take a growth off his leg. He is a gangsta, he tells Andy. He mouths off opinions full of hatred, racist rants against Jews and others. He latches on to Andy. Andy worries: maybe he wants to be my mate. Oh, God. If I'm not his mate, maybe he will come over and slice me up.

The bay has its own dynamic, its own community feelings and fears. Andy becomes intimate with everyone's treatment. He spends a lot of time worrying about the man next to him. His treatment seems to involve having his legs strapped apart so that bone will grow to help his hips and thighs stay together. Andy doesn't quite understand what is going on, but he can see enough to feel very, very sorry for the patient. It looks as if his legs are tied to two ends of a broomstick, like some kind of medieval torture. It is the same with everyone. The doctors come, they draw the curtains round, they have their private conversations with you, they draw the curtains back. Then as soon they go away the other patients start asking: what did he mean by . . . ? You know when he said . . . ?

Andy learns that after operations, many patients feel emotional, hostile and depressed. The gangsta opposite calms down. A warmth develops between him and Andy. They share a few jokes.

One afternoon Andy's old girlfriend and new girlfriend turn up to visit at exactly the same time. There is some embarrassed twitching at the end of the bed. New girlfriend exits. Old girlfriend puts Andy on the rack. Who is she? Where did you meet her? How long have you known her? The gangsta loves it. When she leaves, he leans over with a big grin and asks, 'What was going on there, man?'

When his new friend leaves, Andy gets depressed. Two old and very sick patients are put in the bay. One is a suicide attempt who has thrown himself under a Tube train; the other is disturbed, and talks to himself all through the night, quietly, threateningly, under his breath. Andy cannot sleep. The next morning he pleads quietly with a nurse: can't he be moved to somewhere with younger people? Please? Some stable people? Anywhere but here.

Andy hates the bedpan routine. After the first operation the nurses give him heavy laxatives. I don't want them, he says. The nurses take pity and wheel his bed into the bathroom so he can take a shit in private. He discovers they do it with virtually everyone.

The first bedpan he gets is plastic. The nurses help him up on it in the bathroom, and leave him. He knows immediately that it is no good. He is 15 stone. It starts to buckle under his weight. It is too shallow. If he uses it, he is going to be sitting in his own excrement. They get him another one. He fills it. He hates it. It seems almost bestial and unhygienic. He has got a massive 16-inch wound around his pelvis and he is getting shit everywhere, rolling around in it, almost. What am I? he thinks. What have I become?

Then the nurses come in, breezy and friendly. 'Don't worry, we'll have everything cleaned up in a couple of minutes.' They wipe his bum. Put fresh sheets on the bed. Clean him up. Suddenly as they wheel him back he feels fantastic, warm and clean and safe. Like a baby again. These are great people, he thinks. There is no pretence, no conversational hedging of bets, no verbal obliqueness, just functionality. He feels released.

From then on, he gets into the habit of always asking loudly, 'Steel, please, as deep as you have got.'

9

The windowless room is cluttered with a desk, some filing cabinets and a computer, but has a stale, unused air to it. A fading health-education poster of Superman fighting Nick O'Teen is coming off one wall. A photo of snow-covered chalets decorates the other. The whole room is painted powder blue and split top and bottom by a thick marble-effect dado. It is a room where people talk around their problems, but rarely stay. A quarter of the room is partitioned off by wall and curtain, behind which is a bed and equipment for testing blood pressure. At the desk, Dr Bateman, starting his afternoon out-patients' clinic, opens a thick, brown-foldered sheaf of notes and turns slightly to address the first patient, who sits quietly in an old chair to one side.

'Dr Evans has written to say that you have a cough, it bothers you, I have to look at you and find out why you are coughing. Is that why you think you are here, sir?'

The man nods. He is old, in his late 70s, with rheumy eyes and large, gnarled hands which rest on top of his walking stick in front of him. He was clearly once a big man, but now he is shrunk with age. Only his thick grey hair and the broad belly stretching his dark blue jumper speak of better, more vigorous times. He watches the doctor intently, with a slightly puzzled look on his leathery face, as if he is having difficulty comprehending what is going on.

The physician's tone is courteous but clipped. 'Do you smoke?'

'I haven't smoked for five years. I dropped it just like that,' says the man, clearly astonished at his own willpower. The physician is unimpressed.

'How long have you had the cough?'

'Oh, I've bin coffin' at night and it's bin going on for a period of time.'

'Well, a period of time is a piece of string. Can you be more specific?'

'A matter of weeks, I would say.'

The doctor does not believe him. 'Were you coughing at New Year?'

'No.'

'Easter?'

'Yes.'

'Did anything happen?'

'Not really, it just came on.'

'You didn't have bad flu?'

'No.'

'Is it always the same?'

'Yes.'

'Do you bring up phlegm?'

'Yes.'

'What colour is it?'

'Yellow colour.'

'Been going on since the beginning?'

'Yup.'

'Does it keep you awake?'

'I've noticed that I wake much earlier, at 5 a.m., like.'

'Is it the coughing that wakes you, or something else?'

'Something else.'

'You want to pass water?'

But the patient has lost the thread. 'I've been waiting to have my cataract done. I had one done in my left eye a year ago, now I'm waiting for the right one, and I'm a bit annoyed about it actually. I've been waiting . . .'

Bateman cuts in. 'You had no cough when they did the cataract operation?'

'No.'

'Now, you've already had a chest X-ray at George's, and you had another here in 1994 . . . Are you breathless?'

'No, not really.'

'Pain in the chest?'

'No.'

'When you cough, does it hurt your chest?'

'No.'

'Have you been gaining or losing weight in the last few months?'

'Gainin'.'

'Are your ankles swelling?'

'No.'

'Are you eating too much?'

'Yes.'

'Now, you have a problem with diabetes?'

'I have had it for 20 years, I use insulin.'

'And the diabetic clinic monitors you. Are they happy with your progress?'

'Well, not much progress really.'

Bateman twitches impatiently. He leans forward. 'Is your wife with you, Mr Cunningham?'

'Yeah, she is outside.'

Bateman leaves the room briefly and returns with a short woman, old but alert, dressed in a smart dark sweater and tartan trousers. She sits down, resting her own walking stick against the side of the chair. She listens as her husband answers the physician's questions about diabetes. Then Bateman turns to her. The GP, he says, thinks her husband is taking one type of pills. Her husband say he isn't. Who's right?

'He's not taking them,' she says.

'How much did you used to smoke, Mr Cunningham?'

'About 60 a day.'

'Work?'

'He started as a printer and ended up as SOGAT secretary, retired at 65,' she says. Her foot taps nervously. 'His waterworks have been up the creek as well,' she adds, nodding.

Bateman takes Mr Cunningham into the examination cubicle and asks him to remove his jumper and lie on the bed. He rolls up the man's shirtsleeve and takes his blood pressure, slipping the little black rubber bag over his arm and gently inflating it.

'Swing your legs over the edge of the bed. I want to have a listen to your back,' he says. 'Deep breath, and out. When you were lying down you seemed a bit breathless.'

The wife stares at the poster opposite, her lips pursed. *Help me crush the evil Nick O'Teen!* says Superman, his hands round the villain's throat.

'Do you know what an ECG is?' asks Bateman in the cubicle. 'We need to get one of them done. When did we last do a blood test?'

'I think it was done by the GP,' the wife says.

The man comes back to his seat, pulling his jumper over his head.

'How bad are your waterworks?'

'Cor, something terrible, aren't they, Doris? Terrible.'

'When did it become a problem?'

'At night . . .'

'Do you have to get up at night to pass water? Does it hurt?'

'No . . .'

His wife butts in: 'They can be OK for a week then he wets the bed . . .

'I might be able to help him, give him a diuretic pill to take in the morning. It means he won't be able to go out early on. His blood pressure is too high, there are lots of signs that the heart is working too hard. I will give you some pills that will get you to pass more water during the day. You're going to see a urologist at St Helier? Perhaps I should write to Dr Evans and say it should all be done in one place.'

'Perhaps you could sort out me waterworks, Doctor?'

'I can't do your waterworks. I wouldn't be much good if I tried. It's more sensible if it's all done in one place.'

Bateman spends a long time looking something up in a drug book. 'Come back in two weeks' time. I want to see that my treatment is working, not making you worse. Can you bring all the pills he is on? We'll get you fit yet.'

'Thank you, Doctor,' they both say as they leave. The physician looks at the GP's letter again. The words 'fundholding practice' are embossed at the top. He has spent the last 15 minutes suppressing his anger. An X-ray at one hospital. A urologist at another, then sending the patient into St Thomas' to get his cough looked at. This way and that. What is it all about? Pounds and pence. Those little screws of existence.

'It makes me bloody furious,' Bateman mutters, before going out to see who's next.

10

'I will tell you what happened in the early days of the internal market,' says the professor, leaning across his desk, his eyes dark with intent. He is one of the hospital's most senior specialists, an eminent virologist of Indian descent, with an agile brain, a plummy English upper-class accent and a grace-and-favour flat in Lambeth Palace – a quietly guarded Establishment perk for those at the very top of the St Thomas' tree. He runs the laboratories in North Wing, providing clinical diagnostic services for doctors on the St Thomas' and Guy's sites, and oversees research into cancer and HIV-related viruses.

'We won the contract to provide the laboratory service to the Maudsley Hospital opposite King's, right? It was absolutely crazy. They didn't know who to talk to here if there was a problem, we didn't know the sisters on the wards.' He goes on: you couldn't interpret results in conjunction with colleagues, consultants couldn't pop in and chat about patients, you couldn't easily send junior staff over on an educational basis, they couldn't send people here. The whole idea of providing a better service for patients just went out the window.

He sighs. 'We lost the contract in the end. And you know what? George's won the contract to provide lab services for the psychiatric unit here! Ha!' He laughs bitterly, turning to stare out at the London nightscape behind Parliament. 'Crazy, absolutely crazy. I try to be apolitical, but it's very difficult nowadays.'

11

Andy finds himself looking at Parliament for hours, studying its brown-quarry rhythms. He is getting on well with the nurses, trying to catch the beat of their hospital lives, see who likes who, what entanglements each encounters outside the institution's protective grasp. It's what any patient does. He looks out, he watches in. He watches the ward sister especially closely. She is blonde, assertive, a single mother, capable of dealing with anything. When she comes round with the 'sweet trolley', doling out everyone's drugs, he tries to tease more facts out of her, get her to talk about her personal life, say something about herself. Occasionally she loses herself in the conversation, then she snaps back into professional mode. He finds he watches everyone more closely. Every newcomer to the ward seems interesting. There is so little other stimulation. Some patients have televisions. It irritates him. He hears them but cannot see what is going on.

He gets a whiff of sex occasionally. On one occasion he is taken down for an X-ray by a young doctor, a houseman. He notices the nurses express some surprise about him wanting to accompany Andy. When they reach the X-ray, Andy understands why he was so keen to come along. He too wants to see the radiologist, who is trim and beautiful in a cultured way. The houseman, big and awkward, with a cut-glass accent, makes a fool of himself, too eager to help. At one point he slips on his way to the sink and nearly goes flying, just holding his balance, going beetroot red at his own clumsiness. Andy wonders if he is some kind of upper-class buffoon. It is all so curious, he thinks. Despite the saturation of medical images in the modern-day media, so much of hospital life is still like a Carry On film. Consultants *are* like James Robertson Justice. There *is* bedpan humour. People *do* slip on pools of piss on the floor. The hospital is full of weird characters, like Steve, the porter, who wheels him down for X-rays. He is young, sniffs a lot, and shows a careless disregard for other people's limbs. He pushes the bed so fast that more than once Andy finds unexpected visitors virtually tipped on top of him.

Eventually Andy is moved to a six-bed bay. The other patients are younger and chattier. He finds out more about what is going on in the hospital. Stranded in his bed, immobile for most of the day, he tries to build up a picture of what the rest of the site might be like. Friends bring him cappuccino coffee when they visit. He finds it strangely exciting, knowing that they bought it in the hospital, just by the entrance. He can't believe it. What kind of hospital has such good coffee? Other patients tell him about the wards in the old South Wing. He tries to imagine what they are like: long wide halls lined with ranks of beds along each side, illuminated by deep windows stretching up to the ceiling, almost unchanged since Florence Nightingale approved the specifications. But he cannot work out just where the wards are in the jumble of the hospital's geography. He cannot even envisage the building he is in. He can only understand it from the inside, stuck in its entrails, looking out at its spectacular views, but living with its peeling paint, its broken blinds, its tattered lack of maintenance. He cannot see its skin.

He is happier now. He has mastered the bedpan routine and has slowly begun to enjoy leaving all decisions to others. He realises that he likes being treated just as a body rather than as a complicated, singular person. It is something new, something completely different from life outside.

The morning of his second operation, he is taken down to the operating theatre. Andy feels no fear at all, just excited trepidation. It is the excitement he feels on a plane, my God, we could crash! But it's worth it, and you wouldn't know much about it if something happened. He rationalises it: he cannot walk, he is useless as he is, he has to let them take care of him. They will open him up, sort it out and put him back together. He likes the idea of that, of being fixed.

He is first to be operated on that morning. It will be a long operation, four hours or more. He soaks in the atmosphere as the porter pushes him down the corridor. His heart pounds as if he is a little boy again. Suddenly he is in a movie. The trolley glides past the various theatre doors, he glances in, he sees anaesthetists waiting quietly in their bays, making preparations for their first patient. Pulling on gloves. Checking bottles and lines. The blue pyjamas seem almost like space-station suits. Everything is bright and hard and clean and metal and fresh and ready. All he misses is a soundtrack. He needs music for this scene. He cannot understand why there is no music.

He smiles up at the anaesthetist. She smiles back. She is short and Latin and has the smooth demeanour of a successful businesswoman. She visited him in the ward the day before, to talk him through what she would be doing, and all he noticed was that she had big hair and big jewellery, like a Buenos Aires housewife. Now he feels happy in her hands, as if he is the star. Everyone gives him reassuring smiles. He feels heroic, as if he is the Chosen One.

Then gradually, sharply, the illusion fades. He realises the anaesthetist is flustered. She cannot find his notes. The surgeon walks in in his shirtsleeves. He gives Andy a brief smile.

'Where's John?' he asks the anaesthetist. 'Have you seen him? He said he was going to get the films. I don't know what's happened to him.'

Andy notices the anaesthetist looking at her watch.

'I've got to be at Peter's at 12.30,' she says.

Andy turns his head to her. 'Well, don't rush it!' he says. She smiles tensely at him, then, realising her mistake, laughs reassuringly.

'Of course I won't.'

Andy wakes up in the recovery room. His head throbs, his mouth is dry. He feels sick and uncomfortable. He thinks he is going to throw up. He has to sit up or he is going to choke, but he cannot move. He asks the nurse, a man, if he will lift him.

'No,' he says, 'you've got to stay as you are.'

'But I'm going to be sick!' He is drawling his words, still groggy. Already he hates this nurse, who won't ease his pain, who refuses the simplest request.

Andy looks around. He sees a woman in the bed next to him and there is another woman out of sight, sobbing and crying. The atmosphere is tense and cold. They tell him he must stay till his readings are OK. He just wants to get out, get away from this nurse, get back to his old ward. He realises he is stuck with tubes and pipes. He feels round his body. There are seven in all. Seven tubes going into his body! Three are drainage tubes coming out of the wound on his hip. Saline. Epidural in his back. Catheter up his willy.

When a nurse he knows finally comes down to get him, he moans all the way back to his ward about the man who wouldn't prop him up. 'Yeah, I know, I know,' she says soothingly, 'Everyone says the same about him. He's a real pain.'

Once he is wheeled into the ward, he feels as if he is back in the bosom of his family. He feels everything is being organised for his benefit.

12

Managing in a hospital is a thankless business. You try and balance the books, but no one really wants to make the tough decisions: who doesn't get treated, what doesn't get done. Yet a hospital has to be organised. Whoever funds it – the state, the city, the Church, the patients – someone has to run it. Somebody has to decide what is worth spending and what is worth buying. As no one has yet found a way to value a human life, all calculations get fudged in the end.

Over the centuries, governors, aldermen, freemen, churchmen, administrators, even doctors have tried running hospitals. None has ever been a conspicuous success. In the 20th century, nearly every hospital has been teetering on the verge of bankruptcy at one time or another, whatever system was in vogue at the time (and however much was salted away in its own little ring-fenced fund). The more you try and force hospitals to make money, the more they seem to lose it. The more you order them to put their own house in order, the bigger the mess seems to become. Even when you get the money right, as Matthews has (all efficiency targets met and a surplus made every year), the system still squeezes you till you squeak. They say they might give you less because you are so sharp. It's not fair.

Consequently, to be a middle manager in a modern hospital is to be a small fish swimming against the tide, without friends, travelling furiously to get nowhere, just to stay still. Your bosses keep shrinking the budget, your staff feel under threat, the patients expect ever-higher standards, the politicians denigrate your work. The pressure to find extra funds is incessant, the drive into the private sector remorseless. Some managers get torn apart along the way by bigger fish with sharper teeth.

St Thomas' has had its share of little rip-offs and big swindles, just like any other great hospital. The most recent scandal, an imaginative con involving a fake American air ambulance company which billed St Thomas' in advance for bogus air transfers of non-existent private patients, cost the hospital £519,000. The perpetrator, a 34-year-old conman who had previously been jailed for pretending to be a doctor, paid much of the money back, but the damage was done. Newspapers leapt on the swindle as another example of inept NHS management. The stories didn't mention what happened to the managers involved, but some survived. (Bizarrely, the conman himself later returned to St Thomas' for treatment, accompanied by prison officers. He had insisted; it was the only hospital for him.)

Anyone can get conned, if the con is good enough. But somehow to get conned out of public money looks like pig-ignorant negligence. The reality of everyday life for most other managers, however, is never nearly so exciting.

Gill's room is small but tidy. Stuck up in the surgical directorate portakabin wedged beside the corridor joining the hospital's old and new blocks, it smacks of organisation and purpose. Files line one end, a double desk curls round another, a whiteboard is bolted up next to the door. The whole space, no more than 14 feet by eight, is lit by two skylights. There is a seat for Gill at the desk and another for visitors by the door.

Sometimes, she thinks, you have to be mad to be a hospital manager. Friends roll their eyes. They say: what the health service needs is more doctors, not more managers! Those who have had nursing experience ask: how can you be put in charge of running wards and hiring nurses? You've never done it! No, she replies, but I've got others I can ask about that. What I've got is management nous, which is what you need to run big hospitals these days.

She is young, 27, and good-looking, short, with a wide, appealing face and a blonde bob. The doctors like her because she gets things done. Her peers warm to her because she is good company. Since the departments were organised into groups – acute medicine, surgery, clinical services, tertiary services, women and children, dentistry and dermatology – the *esprit de corps* of the surgery managers has grown tight. Most are women in their late 20s and early 30s. They play the system well. They understand each other and what the job demands. Us against the world! Well, often it is us against the other groups, trying to get the best nurses, desperate to stop others poaching beds, juggling patients on the waiting list to get the best income, fending off complaints, coping with the endless media battering, trying to hit budget. But when it works, it works well.

But right now, in a welter of reorganisation, enforced savings, budget cuts and unfilled vacancies, it is close to not working at all. Gill hits the computer button. It warms up to a slow, flat drone. Twenty-four e-mails wink away at her. Twenty-four little cries of *help!* Help me with this idea, help me with this patient, help me with this complaint, help me with a spare bed, please? She leaves them for later. She has a group meeting to go to and figures to look at.

The figures run over reams of paper. She has annual budget figures down one line, cost so far in the year, how much out. Then the description of what she has to pay for: five consultants on the St Thomas' site, another four at Guy's; some are academic, one works part-time at another hospital. All have junior staff: registrars and house officers. And support staff: secretaries and clerks. Then there are the wards for surgery patients and the nurses to run them. All itemised and budgeted for. Then there is the amount of work brought in, and paid for. The planned operations, and the emergencies that shunt them out of the way.

Right now, the wheels are close to coming off the bus. Most of the money comes from the local purchasing authority, which block-buys everything in advance: local A&E, emergency operations, planned operations, the lot. It's always a notional amount, based on what happened last year, but paid for with real cash. When that has been used up, the planned operations wait for the next financial year. GP fundholders, however, can buy their operating slots with their own cash. Consequently managers are under pressure to bump up patients from GP fundholders as it is extra money on top. Which is what Gill has been doing for a month. She loathes doing it, but she has no choice. She has to try and balance the books if she can. And now she has been told that next year, the purchasing authority is having its money cut by the Government, so it can only buy less. The Trust wants to know where she can make savings.

Sometimes it gets to her. Sometimes she just wants to catch the first train back to Croydon. She has patients on the phone pleading for a slot for their hip operation, crying because their hip hurts so much, begging please, please. She has to say no, because their health authority hasn't purchased enough and they are not clinically urgent. Yet their next-door neighbour, with the same condition, can be done months before them, simply because they are at a different GP. Gill is not political, but she hates the way the fundholding system has been introduced – most managers do. It should have been all or nothing, not this ridiculous two-tier system.

And that's not the only worry. Each authority agreement includes an agreed maximum time on the waiting list – twelve months, eighteen months. If someone waits too long for an operation, the hospital is fined. Then there are the theatre sessions to book. Each operating theatre is booked in three-and-a-half-hour sessions. She has to book and buy in the teams around her surgeons: anaesthetists, nurses, equipment. All of that costs just over £500 per session and has to be organised months in advance. Then there are the training needs. It is a teaching hospital. Young surgeons need to get the right variety of work. The consultants lean on her constantly to come up with suitable operations to get their juniors up the ladder.

Other imponderables pop up all the time. When you get the right operations, you find that a couple of your ward nurses have left and you cannot replace them and you don't have the money left for agency cover. No nurses, no beds, no operations. Or you get the nurses and then Medicine commandeers the beds for an emergency. Patients, purchasers, consultants, nurses – you learn to balance them all adroitly. The medical staff understand once you explain the dynamic to them: if they did any operation they wanted, then they would be overperforming the contract to the extent that they were working for free. That would cause an overspend, which in turn would entail cost savings, and the only costs left to save would be jobs. Principally, their jobs. She thinks they understand now. It is the registrars on rotation she feels sorry for. The whole internal market, especially in London where money is being squeezed, is a nightmare for them.

Do the patients understand? No, because you cannot tell them the truth. You cannot say to them, 'Are you registered with a GP fundholder? Then I suggest you should, pronto.' No, you have to cover it up, and they just think the hospital is being inefficient. But all you are doing is trying to make outgoings match incomings. If the Government wants an internal market, that's what you have to do.

Does it create more bureaucracy? Yes, but so does any change in any system.

Do the market reforms bring benefits? Yes, but just how many is hard to judge.

Have the reforms produced a cost-driven rather than a care-driven service? Pass.

Do the media understand? No, that's why every hospital drama portrays managers as evil, slimy bastards, and every politician pledges to reduce their numbers as if they were an infectious disease.

*   *   *

At the surgery group managers' meeting, in an old room near the Governors' Hall, Gill sits down at the dark end, away from the windows that run along one side. Biscuits are passed round. Coffee is poured. The group clinical director – the surgeons' surgeon – is away, so his secretary sits in, taking notes on what the managers say, underlining what has to be referred back for his attention. There are ten others around the table, seven women and three men, all responsible for running surgery on the Trust's two sites. At the head of the long table sits the clinical operations manager, Gill's boss. He has a droopy moustache that gives him a lugubrious air quite at odds with his cheery demeanour. 'Morning, one and all,' he says, kicking the meeting off.

First up is the current round of negotiations over the purchasing requirements of Lambeth, Southwark and Lewisham, the local health authority that is always squeezed for cash. 'Right, the LSL contract restrictions: LSL have broadly accepted that they have got to purchase their version four volume if they are to maintain 18 months' waiting time.' The ten managers stare fixedly ahead, making their own calculations. Some stir their coffee slowly. The negotiations have taken months; everyone is feeling tense about their outcome. To make it worse, the medical school has also discovered that it is to get £2.5m less from the higher education authorities, meaning that some academic posts may go. And a Labour government has pledged to reduce the number of managers in the NHS. Everyone has their own thoughts this morning, but most of the thoughts are about jobs.

'Merton, Sutton and Wandsworth have found some additional pennies to put into their purchasing intentions . . .' The clinical operations manager describes where the cash has come from – the sum set aside for keeping a hypothetical baby in ITU for a year. That is how health authorities work, in hypotheticals. They toss a few ideas in the air, look at what they did last year, and jump. If a baby needs intensive care for 12 months in the next financial year, this time they won't have budgeted for it. Some eyebrows go up. They are used to all this now. One manager, heavily pregnant, looks intently at the sheet of minutes in front of her. Her boss has slipped into management jargon, the drone falls over the room like a light mist: 'The Bromley position is better than expected, City and Hackney have to purchase some elective surgery to keep up the tertiary ratio . . .' Outsiders are suspicious of hospital managers because they don't understand what they do, except make work for themselves. But good managers cope with whatever system is thrown at them. Ask any hospital doctor: they would give their eye teeth for a good manager.

They talk waiting-list times – 'Bromley is uncomfortable about slipping to 18 months' – and shortfalls. There is a gap in the budget of up to £800,000, and the Trust's financial director wants to hear some radical cost-saving suggestions. Already the bureaucracy is tumbling over itself to convince people that this is serious, this is the big one. Some neurologists have been double-warned, in letters from the Trust and, a day later, the medical school. No wonder most in the hospital are tense. 'I think they got the message, there,' says one manager, drolly.

They move on to cost-benefit analyses. They drink more coffee. Behind the operations manager's head an antique clock hangs on the wall, stuck fast on seven past seven. One manager wants to close a ward to save money. The others hum and haw. It's a question of who's paying for what.

'I'm still unhappy with surgical group overspending as a result of the fact that Medicine has people in surgical beds.'

'If you've got someone in A&E who needs to be admitted and a surgical patient can be cancelled, fine, but that doesn't help you with your overspend.'

'I agreed that we would recharge for outliers. If Medicine is occupying surgical beds then we will recharge each other, so at least we don't suffer the consequences.'

'We did recharge beds at Guy's but that was abandoned. Can anyone remember why?'

They all agree they will try and find out. Inevitably, the

group system encourages competition. The operations manager runs through the figures for the other groups. 'Medicine is underperforming by £880,000, Tertiary is overperforming by £1m, Dental and Dermatology is out by £200,000.' The figures wash over them like a soothing balm. Only Surgery is on course, poised to hit the targets it submitted a year before. 'The only people managing their contracts properly are us. You can pat yourselves on the back,' says the manager. His voice carries a faint nasal twang.

Gill talks about Thomas Guy House, the new hospital block built at Guy's. It has been a running disaster ever since it was commissioned. There have been cost overruns and rows with the contractors over fitting out. Little of what it was originally designed for, ten or more years before, is now going into the building. But soon it will be open and Surgery will be using it for planned care. Gill has been round.

'Did you manage to find your way out?'

'Just,' she smiles. No one knows whether a long-running disaster like Thomas Guy House will eventually be a glorious success. At the moment it is still safe to laugh about it.

'Apparently,' she goes on, 'I am going to be trained to take people around. The problem is I cannot get all my consultants together at once, and I don't really want everyone to know that I take people round, otherwise I will be spending all my time there.' The surgeons, it seems, still haven't quite twigged that the move is imminent. She says she has had just one query, as to whether the place will be large enough to perform hand surgery. The managers ponder this for a while.

The urologists have queried the fittings. There are three-room, four-room and five-room options. The architects will still not give any indication as to final prices for fittings. Gill has to decide where to put telephone points. In the end, much of life comes down to this, knowing that wherever you choose to put them it will be wrong. But you struggle on.

They talk nurses. It is the single biggest problem facing the hospital. The retention rate is abysmal and recruitment is tough. Demographics and working conditions are against them. Young nurses will work in the city, go travelling, get married, settle down and look to go back into nursing outside London. Who needs the pressure of a big teaching hospital? Who needs the dangerous travelling, the rotten hours, the grim digs, the stroppy, seriously sick patients, when you can work in a district general hospital for more or less the same money with routine patients in for routine operations in a nicer place with nicer people? The managers don't blame them. They can't pay them more than the national rate because the nursing unions will not allow local pay bargaining. So they are stuck. The shortage has a knock-back effect on everything: beds, operations, other staff. Every year they know they are going to need more beds at the beginning of winter because of the annual flu epidemic. Every year they struggle to sort it out. Last winter it happened again. The medical emergencies had to be put in the beds reserved for surgical patients, the surgery group couldn't admit their planned care operations, the waiting lists got longer, the income got dented, the media started sniffing around. Managers, like doctors, have come to dread the annual winter crisis.

'We've 50 per cent overspent our recruitment budget already.'

'Why don't we push it over properly with some glossy full-page ads?'

'Do they work?'

'I'm willing to go to South Africa and Australia to interview some overseas candidates . . .'

They laugh, but it is no joke. Recruitment from overseas is now an easier option than hiring at home. The managers also know that they can save up to £1,000 a post if they get the recruits themselves, rather than paying an agency. More than five recruits and you've swiftly paid for the trip. Yet equally they know it would be disastrous in PR terms if they were to be seen swanning off to hot places, looking for nurses. Imagine what the *Evening Standard* would make of it. Imagine what the *Sun* would make of it. No one really likes hospital managers, not even other health-service staff. They mistrust them. The managers live with that all the time.

Already they are considering whole ward closures because they have neither the money nor the nurses to run them. Jane, sitting opposite Gill, sighs. How do they tell the nurses who are left? 'If we close it, I don't want want the nursing staff hearing about it from the consultants,' she says, with a faint West Country burr in her accent. She suggests merging two wards, combining the nursing staff, freeing up some money to bring some decent curtains and stuff like that over – 'not megabucks, just a couple of K . . .'

'I've got a cunning plan,' says the operations manager.

'What? Let's all go on holiday and forget it?'

'Yes.'

They all smile. If they could just get a grip on the wards . . .

13

Andy is getting a lot of injections before and after the operations. Stuff going in, stuff coming out. Anti-blood clotting, blood testing. He gets used to it, ward life as a pin-cushion. He watches the cannulae pop his skin for drips and drains with barely a flinch. Soon he is observing his body as dispassionately as the professionals. Go on, put another tap in, he says. A nurse wants to stick a cannula into his wrist. Another nurse is having trouble getting it in. Andy says, put a bigger one in. Go on. It's got to be more useful, he thinks, you can run more things in. He loves the idea that he can see his body as a machine. He is slipping into hospital-think fast.

The catheter pulls him round. He hates it. When he wakes

up from the second operation he cannot believe what they have done, stuck a green rubber tube up his cock. The nurses explain it to him. It has a small bag on the end. When it is inserted into his bladder, they can fill the bag with water and stop it coming out. Please take it out, he begs, please. He feels sore and violated.

He pleads with the nurses till midnight. They tell him they cannot take it out. The consultant will be furious. It cannot come out till he has 'opened his bowels'.

'I'm not going to have a problem doing that. Just take it out. *Please!*'

'If you can't open your bowels, or can't urinate, we will have to put it back in.'

'Don't worry. I'll take that risk.'

'If we have to put it back in and you've a full bladder, it's really unpleasant.'

The nurse looks at him long and hard.

He shakes his head. 'I just want it out,' he says.

Eventually she agrees to take it out.

She draws the tube slowly out of his penis. As it rubs reluctantly out, like a dead worm, his face creases into agony. 'ARGH!' he cries. 'It huuurts!' He feels like a 12-year-old and sees a look of intolerant disapproval flash across the nurse's face.

As the hours tick by, he begins to panic. He wants to urinate, but nothing will come out. His bladder feels strange, scarred. He thinks: oh, God, they are going to stick it back in. Oh, God.

Then he realises he hasn't drunk anything. He must drink as much as possible. Of course, his bladder is empty. He gulps tea and water. It still takes hours but a trickle comes through, then a torrent. He has never been so pleased to see his own piss.

The effect of the catheter lasts for longer than he expects. It is a month before he can no longer feel its intrusion in his flesh. He feels emasculated.

The operation is a success. He is held together with bolts but he feels his flesh firming and mobility returning. Soon after, he hankers to get out. He has to see an occupational therapist, and convince her that he can look after himself. He lies in bed thinking, how quickly can I get out? If I can persuade them to take the first stitches out on Tuesday, then maybe they can take the next stitches out on Friday. That same day I could make sure they find crutches for me, and I could do the various tests . . .

The one thing that keeps him in good spirits is the challenge: he wants to be the fastest-mended person ever. That is all he is interested in. He focuses himself, pulling himself about on his monkey pull, trying to keep moving, working on his muscles.

When he first gets up, after three weeks, he nearly falls over with dizziness as the blood rushes from his head. He has watched others do the same as they master their crutches, and he has vowed, it won't happen to him. But it does. He has been on crutches in the past, he knows how to use them. But it takes time.

He reads magazines, grimly depressing, filling his time. A friend brings him some marking. 'Anything to keep me busy,' he said to him on the phone, so he can't blame him. Another friend has tracked down his bike, and got it taken to a garage. The garage says it should be written off.

After three and a half weeks, they say he can go, so he packs up his belongings and waits for a friend to drive him home. He says goodbye to the staff and the patients. Some look envious to see him go. He thinks he may miss the hospital. He knows that twenty years ago he would have been crippled. Now he is walking out. Great place, he thinks, great people to do what they do.

14

Gill went into management because she thought it was a good career. She was brought up in south London, where she still lives. Her parents were teachers. She got A levels in politics, English and sociology, and a degree in social administration – the kind of degree you get if you want to work in the public sector, the probation service, say, or in social work. After university she went to Australia for a bit, then came back and applied for every job she could see in the *Guardian* for three months. It was just after the Gulf War and the job market was slack. But persistence paid off. Eventually she got a post with Greenwich Health Authority, in their commissioning department. She did that for 18 months and then moved to another authority in south London. Her job was to buy services for the population. She moved again, and this time she was buying off the Guy's and St Thomas' Trust. She liked the bustle and faded glamour of the big hospitals, the chance to get involved in operational management as opposed to just pushing figures around. When she heard a job was going in the surgery group, she talked her way in.

She knew what to expect: after all, she had been buying off the Trust in her last job. She knew the reputation for clinical excellence was high, certainly with the local population, who would always rather go to Thomas' or Guy's if given the chance. They simply believed there were better doctors there. But in fact you only find out who the good doctors are by working in a place. She also knew of Thomas' other reputation: for posh medical students and nurses in Alice bands, twin-sets and pearls, whose daddies practised out of rooms in Harley Street. There was a bit of that left, but not much. Thomas', she thought, was probably stuffier than Guy's, a bit more formal and less down to earth. At Guy's everyone seemed to know each other better, they had been working there together for years. At Thomas', somehow, there were still invisible barriers everywhere, between consultants, managers and workers. The typical Thomas' response, if you wanted to get anything done quick, was 'Sorry, I can't do that, love, not without permission.'

But the managers were young, there was little dead wood – not like you would find out in the sticks – and there was no culture of macho management, as in some other London hospitals. People had their gripes, but if they looked at other hospitals outside London they would see this place was quite well run. That's how it looked from the inside, anyway.

'Right, one thing they are concerned about is the Continuum of Care thing.'

'Anyone read it?'

'No, it's too long.'

They all sigh. There is a lot to get through. The operations manager is going round the table to see if anyone has anything else they want to discuss.

'There's a protocol being written about needle-stick injuries to staff handling patients. I'm hoping to meet with David about this one. There are all sorts of issues going on.'

No one is sure what the Department of Health guidelines are on the matter. The problem is how to tell if the patients involved are HIV positive. You cannot test them without their consent.

'They will test and test again in three months. If any risk, going to suggest prophylactic AZT within two hours. But it's all very hazy and unclear.'

'There are a lot of anaesthetists who have needle-stick injuries who just don't bother to report it.'

'Yes, well, it happened to a long-term agency staff the other week. The thing that panicked the staff was that when they went to Occupational Health they started talking about AZT.

The long-term effect of that is not nice: nausea, night sweats. Luckily the patient involved recognised the staff concern and agreed to immediate screening. But we couldn't get hold of any counselling.'

'And what if the patient is just coming out of theatre? They can't give consent. What's the implication for the patients?'

A hush falls on the room for the first time.

'I'd be interested to know what Charles thinks of this,' says the operations manager, looking pointedly at the surgeon's secretary. She nods, scribbling away furiously. Another manager intercedes.

'Infection Control say we are the first trust to roll with this.'

They move on. Each manager details the beds he or she is likely to lose in both hospitals because of staff shortages. One is closing beds on Queen's Ward, another on Aston. A third is going out to sell the hospital's services to GPs and wants to take some clinical directors with her, to address specific issues.

Finally they look at a report of what came up at the last surgeons' meeting. There is worry about the amount of staff now wearing surgical gear – the operating bibs called theatre greens – out on the wards. More worrying, some doctors might be returning to operate without changing their greens, bringing into the theatre whatever bacteria they might have picked up on the way.

'The problem is that there are so many people who have to wear them, there is no control over who can wear them and who can't. To control it, we would have to have people on every exit, making staff sign them in and out. Who's going to pay for that?'

'And lots of the doctors do it, it's not just the juniors. If they see consultants doing it, you can't blame them.'

'And it's not the ones who turn up to the surgeons' committee who do it.'

The operations manager places his hands flat on the table. 'I'll have a word with the medical director,' he says. 'It might come to making it a disciplinary offence.'

'It's not just wearing the clothes out of the theatres,' says another, leaning forward. 'There are surgeons who think it is macho to walk around with *blood* all over their greens. That's the sort of thing we are up against.'

'You know what it is,' says a woman down the end. 'It's the *ER* culture. They think it looks good. They think, hey, let's all walk around in our pyjamas. It's cool.'

We live in a culture of complaint. Gill sees it first-hand. She spends about a day a week just working through the complaints that come in about her department. She makes the right enquiries, writes the right responses. Some complaints are more complicated than they appear. She had one on her desk from a GP criticising the way a patient was handled on one of her wards. She didn't blame the GP, the patient had been insistent. But when she checked with the nursing staff she found the patient had given them two thank-you cards and two boxes of chocolates on leaving. Only later did she decide she was upset. It turned out she was a schizophrenic.

Other complaints roll on for years. One she is still dealing with dates back to 1993, when a patient operated upon at Guy's appeared to catch MRSA from the hospital. Methicillin-resistant staphyllococcus aureus is one of those things that people in hospitals try not to talk about. Like the animal house at Thomas', where the animals used in research are kept (everyone knows what floor they are on, but most like to pretend it's a secret, for fear of alerting animal-rights activists, who know everything anyway). Similarly MRSA, a debilitating infection picked up from bacteria in operating theatres and hospital wards, is not something that is openly discussed very much. However, it is, by some judgements, rampant throughout hospitals and nursing homes in the south of England. Anyone undergoing an operation which exposes bone is particularly vulnerable to it. Patients succumbing to it are swiftly put into side rooms and 'barrier nursed'. It is as bad as it sounds.

Occasionally the press or a documentary-maker will run with an MRSA story, but most leave it alone. Hospitals just live with it. They don't talk about it because they don't want to frighten the patients. They don't want to look like germ factories. They don't want business to drop off.

On Gill's desk sits a fat file, inches thick, concerning a hip-replacement patient who did appear to get MRSA. The complaint is now being handled by the community health council, a sort of up-and-at-'em Citizens' Advice Bureau for angry patients. Gill has had to answer all the questions. Was MRSA prevalent in the hospital at the time? Why was the patient put on that ward on that day? Was the patient the only one on the operating list that day? Did the patient go in first or last? (You have less chance of getting MRSA if you are first in.) Getting the responses together has taken weeks. It all happened four years ago. The staff have changed. The doctor who performed the operation has left.

Then there are the staff complaints. There was a young man, gunshot wound in the leg, causing hell on a ward, abusing the nurses, intimidating the other patients, coming on like a gangster. All day he would have his posse of friends around him, backing him up, taking calls on their mobile phones, scaring anyone who came past. The ward sister talked to him but he took no notice. So Gill went over with Eileen, her number two. They called up security and met the sister outside the ward. She thought the security staff would just make the situation worse. So Gill and Eileen went in on their own. Eileen, who is bigger and older than Gill, laid down the law. 'You,' she said, pointing at the friends, 'no more mobile phone calls or you're out. You,' she said, turning to the patient, 'no more than three friends at any time. Those are the rules. And BEHAVE.' Then they talked to him a bit. It turned out he was just a frightened boy. Frightened that he was going to lose his leg. Frightened that someone was going to come back and finish off the job. He wanted his friends round him for protection. You couldn't blame him.

Does she need all that hassle? Well, she likes the variety. She reckons she gets pretty well paid, over £25,000, for doing what she enjoys. But there are niggles. A friend asked her the other day: what's your budget?

Around £6.8m plus £2m of this, that and the other.

Monkeys and peanuts, he sniffed.

Which meant?

If she was in a major multinational business running that type of budget, she would get paid far more.

But she said: I like doing this. The hours are OK. I am working late at the moment but that's because of the funding crisis and sorting out what the purchasers are going to pay next year. But generally I can fit everything in between nine and six. I like the unexpected nature of it, I like the core management aspect too, the staff difficulties, the disciplinary problems, the patients ringing up, the people asking for protocols for strategic documents, the different doctors – professionals who you would never really get to speak to if you were just an ordinary lay person. Doctors with huge resources of knowledge built up over decades, leaders in their field.

The budget stuff? Well, she can handle it. Numeracy isn't her strength but she can crunch the numbers. No, what you really need for her job is tact, diplomacy and discretion. That gets you through far more. You have to think of the effect of everything you do. So often in the hospital you hear people saying, 'No one told *me*.' Everything you do as a manager has huge implications for people.

And politics? She doesn't talk politics really. Whichever political party is in power will run the NHS how they want. The capital investment is a gripe. Like the London Underground, you can run the NHS with as little money as possible, but soon everything starts falling apart. But if she was in charge, the first thing she would do is wipe out the difference between fundholding and non-fundholding GPs. Then the difference between resources in the city and in the shires. Then sort out some money to do the older hospitals up. Then ... maybe she does talk politics occasionally.

15

A fire breaks out one night in an empty ward on the twelfth floor of North Wing. Forty patients are evacuated safely. The fire brigade soon have the situation under control. Tee is dragged from bed at half past midnight to handle the irate press. 'This is no good,' the *Sun* reporter shouts at him. 'Where are the flames?' God, what it takes to make them happy, thinks Tee.

16

The doctor leans back in his chair. He is young, barely in his mid-30s, stocky, with brown hair clipped short above dark eyes and an aquiline nose. Born in London but trained in Edinburgh, he still carries a trace of a well-spoken Scottish accent. He is wearing a shirt, tie, chinos and loafers. On the desk in front of him lie a sprawl of medical books, a sheaf of loose paper and two fat CVs. His computer, an Apple Mac, hums quietly beside him. The room is windowless, small – barely big enough for two – and airless, squeezed into the heart of the medical department on the fifth floor of Thomas' North Wing. Parts of the corridor look as if a bomb has just gone off. Fat black wires hang out of holes in the roof panelling. The doctor keeps the door open so he can breathe.

The CVs are his. He is unhappy and wants to leave. He has an interview for a post at another London hospital in a week's time. As a senior registrar, he has gone about as far as you can go before becoming a consultant. He has been offered a job to stay at Thomas' but is depressed at what is happening at the hospital. It is not so much the way the Trust is run as the role of the academic side of the hospital, which he feels is making it increasingly difficult for those doctors who want to concentrate on the clinical side. Even though he has a sparkling academic record – his CV is 24 pages thick, bristling with prizes won, lectures given, research experience gained – he feels he is being sucked into a grinding university bureaucracy. He is one of the casualties of the growing tension between the hospital's two roles: curing and teaching. The teaching side, which involves academic research, holds power over too many appointments. He hates the internal politics that generates, common to so many university bureaucracies. He just wants to be a proper doctor.

His views are not simply of the left or right, just pragmatic, like most doctors. He is basically pro-Trust, and pro-internal market, but against what he sees as the increasing academic grip on the hospital. He speaks with the fluency of an accomplished lecturer, underpinned by the frustration of someone who feels he has been banging his head against the ceiling for too long. His words tumble out unchecked.

'I've been a senior registrar with the two chest firms at Guy's and Thomas' for four years. I am accredited in general medicine, respiratory medicine, and allergy and clinical immunology, that's triple accreditation, and I have an academic profile as well, my lecturing. That's not so much teaching but researching. You've got to remember that what you are seeing here is the merger of clinical and academic services. You only see it in the large teaching hospitals. I do teaching too. There's bedside clinical teaching for undergraduate and postgraduate students. Then seminar tutorials and postgraduate teaching too. In the last year and a half I have been spending 75 per cent of my time looking after patients, 15 per cent on research and 10 per cent on teaching. Two years ago I would have been spending 80% of time on research.'

'It's like the army here, it's as regimented as that. The chain of command rests on the consultant. In the past the consultant used to choose his own team, but now the senior registrar is a regional appointment. Yet if a consultant tells a registrar to do something, he will do it. That is the way it goes. Responsibility flows in the opposite direction. The more senior you get the less time you actually spend on the wards with patients. I have care of patients in A&E and out-patients and on wards, and as well as those clinical responsibilities I do practical techniques like bronchoscopies. In addition to that, I've got a pastoral care role to make sure that everyone on the team is happy, there are no conflicts of personalities. I organise the holiday arrangements, ensuring not too many people are away at any one time, and stuff like that.

'St Thomas' is still very prestigious. It has a reputation for being hoity-toity. It's changing now, but you notice that all the nurses are doctors' and dentists' daughters, or nice shire ladies. It's very much an upper-middle-class hospital, and that's reflected in the traditions: there's a good social life, good dinners. The trimmings are great. You have a summer ball, a Christmas dinner. It's all army terminology: the doctors' common room is called the mess; there are mess dinners every three months, which are black-tie with plenty of booze. Everything is subsidised, either from the consultants' own pockets or from donations. It's the same in a lot of hospitals, but it's much more stylish here, and a bit of style is nice sometimes. For junior doctors it can be fun. There are lots of parties, house officers change every three months and you tend to go out a lot. It's very much an army-based mentality. When you work, you work, and in junior years it is quite traumatic because you are not accustomed to seeing what they see, but eventually you get desensitised. You work hard, and you play hard.

'But I am getting out. I was offered another job here but I've decided not to take it. It was an academic appointment. What's happening here – and it will get worse when King's merges with UMDS, the medical school here – is that the hospital is being taken over by medical bureaucrats. The real power is in the medical school. Thomas' may be the main provider of acute services for the Trust, but who is appointed to provide those services is going to be a decision of the medical school, and it's full of academic bureaucrats, with a major civil-service mentality. If you just want to do medicine, where do you stand? I have a prestigious academic profile but I want to be a clinician. I do not want to spend more and more of my time pushing paper around, trying to become more powerful in the institution. I would like to spend four days a week doing clinical work and one day a week doing private practice and getting on with the rest of my life.

'Here it's very competitive, very nitpicking, very backbiting, with a lot of politics involved in it. The appointments are controlled by academics. These academics are not interested in the clinical side. What they want to do is get rid of the clinical side, but they know they need clinical patients to exist. Look at Harvard Medical School. There is no hospital at Harvard. Harvard has contracts with other hospitals, but not on the Harvard site. Here the animosity between academics and clinicians is intense. Academics think clinicians are a waste of space. Clinicians think academics do nothing. Clinicians do work you can gauge. A lot of academic work is just being done so you can be seen to be doing it. It may make you powerful in the institution but at the end of the day it doesn't make you feel that you have done a good day's work. Thomas' doesn't exist on its own any more. It has been swamped by the academic. The hospital is here on sufferance now to provide raw material for our medical students.

'The big conflict in hospitals now is in the larger teaching hospitals, and it's between academics and clinicians. Academics view the Trust as a source of patients for students and biological samples for doing research. The Trust looks on the medical school with terror because it knows that is where power is going to be. It really doesn't matter to UMDS how the clinical services are going. Some heads of department are completely uninterested, they just like to have access to patients for clinical trials. Come back in 10 years' time. You will have a proliferation of private doctors, private hospitals and a private tier of medicine. Teaching hospitals will become massive academic institutions only doing complicated or interesting work, and in order to become a consultant you will have to be willing to spend most of your life in the institution.'

He shrugs and packs up his papers before heading across to the student bar.

17

In the sandwich queue at Tommy's Deli near the out-patients' reception, Gill plans out her afternoon. There's another managers' meeting, informal, over sandwiches, to look at the various bed-closure plans in more detail. Then she has to squeeze on to the shuttle bus to Guy's and sit in on interviews for a new ward sister. Three applicants, 40 minutes each, three of them on the panel: a consultant, a senior sister and Gill. Generally she asks the same questions: what would you do if someone couldn't do the job? What would you do if someone kept calling in sick but never brought in a sick note? How would you juggle the beds if you had got too many patients waiting? That's what being a sister is all about nowadays: people issues, bureaucracy.

The sandwich queue is long and getting longer by the minute. By one o'clock it will be about 30 people long. You either buy here or go to the open-plan cafeteria in the Lambeth Wing. Most of the staff prefer to eat on the hoof, which means joining the queue, or buying sandwiches from the newsagent. The light in the north-facing foyer is muted. People sit around, quiet, depressed, waiting for their prescriptions from the pharmacy opposite or just killing time before an appointment. The deli queue snakes out around the pillars in the main thoroughfare, getting in everyone's way. Gill takes orders for friends, a sandwich for another manager, a roll for one of the Surgery registrars. Three men in silly paper hats take the orders behind the counter and slap the fillings on bread with the sort of weary concentration that a temporary job demands. They do people a favour by spreading the fillings generously. Today's special is coleslaw and bacon. The coleslaw is too tart and the bacon pieces underdone.

Gill distributes what she has bought and carries her sandwich and drink up to the meeting room in the corridor behind her office. Ten institution chairs circle the small room. The executives drift in. All were at the management meeting in the morning. Tony, the operations manager, is already ensconced, file on lap, blue blazer over the back of his chair. A younger man, skinny, with a big smile and glasses, has arrived with a sheaf of financial data. The managers sit around, picking at their sandwiches while their boss talks.

'I thought it would be worth getting us together to talk about the suggestions with regard to beds, theatres and so on.' Tony rambles slightly, discussing the options for saving money in the forthcoming year. The discussion broadens. They all move swiftly into their own jargon, painless managerial shorthand for the cuts proposed. Such and such saves us 230K. Closing Sarah and having a hotel is 160K. Elected activity is down by 10 per cent.

'Well,' says Tony, 'we said let's look at increasing occupancy by 5 per cent, and that enables us to close 26 beds. I don't feel particularly strongly about closing a ward. I certainly don't want to force through a wider closure if there is a more sensible plan.'

Is it enough? Twenty-six beds? The sandwich bags rustle. The woman opposite Tony puts down her roll and leans forward.

'I think a lot of variable income comes in from the Guy's end from their outreach clinics. Let's find out how much first. Because through Sarah you get outliers and gynae. If we are going to close some beds they are going to have to be cut more fairly than our rather crude proposal of just shutting Sarah.'

Another woman in the corner, drinking from a small bottle of mineral water, nods in agreement. 'The only other option would be to transfer some in-patient sessions to day-patients. We would have to recover them in the wards ...'

'That's quite a problem,' says a third. 'I can't fit any more day-patients in.'

Andrew, the data man, shuffles his papers. 'LSL said 35 per cent day-cases, and that's what they are purchasing.'

'If they want to argue for a day-case rate that we can't deliver, well, I'm sorry, I can't sign a contract on that basis,' says Tony, shaking his head.

What about theatres? There's only one theatre available for the work, so that's only 10 sessions. They do the arithmetic. 'The only possibility is to move sessions from here to Lewisham ...'

Tony sighs. 'We've got to have a mix of elective, in terms of day-cases and in-patients, at a rate that will allow us to deliver the 18 months' maximum waiting. We need to crunch the numbers.'

The data man nods, and promises to get the correct figures to the directorate managers. Some of them look at him rather wearily. The atmosphere in the room thickens as a pensive fug envelopes them.

'Let's say we only have 13 beds we don't need,' continues Tony. 'Is it worth taking out half a ward? What else can we do with them?'

'My concern is how we do it,' says the woman opposite. 'Beds will have to come out, it's only a question of how. I don't think we should ring-fence beds for variable income. No way that we can bring hernias and cysts and crap in while we have got patients piling up in A&E that happen to be contracts.'

'And quite rightly the clinicians say even if we get fined £5,000 for the 18-months-late patients, how can we morally not treat the urgents?'

'I think you can if you have got a dedicated list.'

'But I've got pages of oesophageal cancers waiting to come in!'

There is a pause.

'You're looking at me as if I've got two heads or something.'

'I was just thinking,' smiles Tony, 'that this MSC course is obviously making you more principled.'

They all grin, then take turns to throw their own suggestions in.

'Would the clinicians be more comfortable with us not doing the GPF stuff till we've cleared off lots of the urgent stuff?'

'Some weeks there isn't too much urgent and we can whisk in the variable income.'

'If we stick with the 13-bed scenario: do we really want to take them out? Or do we want to use them to bring occupancy levels down? We'll still have those beds in place – so long as we don't fill them up with stuff we don't want.'

'If a bed is there we will fill it. They always get used.'

'I am going to have a slight backlog of electives.'

'Can you not bring your 18-monthers in as 16 months?'

'I will end up with too few beds for emergency and trauma. It will improve if I can get some nurses . . .'

'What about the bed losses at St Thomas'? We have said the beds to go will be day beds. Take six off Nightingale and the remainder off Sarah.'

'What about the nurses? Can we use them elsewhere?'

'It's a case of where the nurses want to go. If there are vacancies elsewhere then they can go there. We can't force them to go to Orthopaedics!'

Tony asks round the room if anyone can afford to lose any nurses. No one can. Maybe, he says, they should look at it another way. Perhaps they can save money by attacking cost overruns in the theatres. The problem, he says, is created by those surgeons who are habitually late in starting. They all nod. Another manager takes up the theme.

'We just shouldn't allow these people to roll in an hour and a half late,' he says. 'We have to pay people to sit around twiddling their thumbs waiting for them to arrive and then pay them overtime when it runs over. It's bad management.'

'The other issue is people coming in on time but still running over. Then we have to ask: are the right operations appearing on the list? If we have people regularly overrunning then we ought to be giving them an additional list between nine and five and thus lose the overtime payments.'

A couple of the managers are looking down at their shoes, deep in thought. There is a nervous cough.

'Mike has calculated a new index called an inefficiency index. And the most common inefficiency is underrunning.'

'That's because we haven't got enough beds to put patients in!' says a woman who has been engrossed in her sandwich till now.

'Talking of beds, is ENT and Plastics still merging?'

Tony purses his lips. No one seems to know. As the data man hands round more sheets of figures, one of the women managers pulls a face theatrically behind his back. Gill grins. They quibble over the figures and Tony beams as he pulls out another inconsistency in the data.

'You can't bullshit a bullshitter,' he says, as he looks around the room.

18

When he was a young boy, Tony Young saw at first hand just what the hospital could do for people. His mother, who had pulmonary tuberculosis and attended St Thomas' for treatment, often used to bring him with her. It was before antibiotics for TB had been discovered, and from the age of six he became quite accustomed to watching his mother go through the complex procedure of having her lungs collapsed deliberately, in order that they could rest. It was achieved by inserting large needles into her chest, and putting air in between the chest wall and the lung. It was all a bit of a performance, with the doctor getting out his box of needles and making a show of it. What effect would that have on a boy, watching your mother murdered and reborn so often? It didn't put him off, anyway. He was fascinated by medical procedure from an early age.

Yet being a doctor was not his first choice. He wanted to be an architect, and his father said fine, if you want to, but if you are a doctor and like being a doctor, then you can do that all the time. If you are an architect, then you might get frustrated because you are not allowed to build the buildings you want. By such persuasions are doctors made. So Young followed his father's advice, and pursued his interests in his own time, painting and studying fine arts. In these ways prospective doctors have been eased into medicine for generations, many of them just doing it because there is a family connection. And the system conspires to pull them in. You don't have to sit on a selection panel for more than 10 minutes to realise that most doctors prefer candidates from medical families. It is never discussed or acknowledged – because employment laws prohibit such preference being exercised – but every doctor knows the score. Coming from a medical family means you have a better grasp of what you are letting yourself in for. It's like marrying another doctor: you know what to expect. You know your spouse is there for the patients when he or she isn't there for your own family. You know the demands of the job. Choosing doctors' kids, to many of the senior staff, is just a bit of clonal selection. The older teaching hospitals like St Thomas' in the past operated that way for years; it was one of their defining characteristics. Doctors' kids might not make the brightest doctors but, as Young likes to point out, whoever said medicine was the place for a first-class brain?

*   *   *

The students are two tall boys and a nervous, keen girl. All three look barely out of puberty. If the medical director said BOO they would probably drop dead with shock, so tightly are they holding themselves. It is quite understandable: a session with the hospital's most powerful doctor is not one you would want to fluff.

They are waiting for him in an old Nightingale ward for general surgical patients. The place appears cavernous after the modern bay wards elsewhere in the hospital. Forty metres in length, with 12 to 14 beds on each side, long windows and awkwardly placed central stations made up of old desks and filing cabinets. They cannot stand in the middle for long without getting in someone's way: the meal trolley, a shuffling patient, a pair of nurses, another doctor with his students. Twenty-odd pairs of patient eyes watch them as they walk around, gauging their purpose, their use, their status. Here, unlike in most of the other wards, where patients are pegged out flat, seriously ill, the occupants of the beds sit up, watching keenly, some half getting up, maybe going for a walk, with inquisitive hope in their eyes. Faced with this wall of scrutiny, the students cluster and look around nervously, prepared to follow whoever makes the first move, like little white goslings waiting for their gander.

Young sweeps in, white hair, white coat, brisk in pace. He has added a long, red-rubbered stethoscope to his kit. The stethoscope clings to his neck, dangling down to his flies, swinging awkwardly. Perhaps it is the Biggest Swinging Stethoscope in the hospital, or perhaps it is just regulation issue. But the sight of it is not lost on the students. They gather round him as he flicks through some hand-written notes on a filing cabinet. Behind them another doctor is sitting quietly at the bottom of a patient's bed, both hands on one of the patient's feet, gently exercising it, squeezing it, rubbing it. The man wants to walk. The doctor says wait. 'I don't think we can be sure yet, perhaps when the swelling goes down. I know you are bored.' It appears almost as if he is caressing the foot delicately, in supplication, in adoration.

Five beds down, on the other side of the ward, sits a yellow man. He is tall and old, in his sixties perhaps, with a tomahawk face, unbrushed, upright hair and an indented nose. A pair of stripy pyjamas cover his broad body, now knobbly with age like a sack of potatoes and sagging slightly under its loose skin. Those patches of his body that are visible – his head, a bit of chest, long feet with gristly nails – reveal his condition. From head to foot he is covered in large patches of vivid yellow ochre, as if someone has indiscriminately decided to decorate the bits of him that aren't already flushed bright pink. And it's a deep-down yellow, coming up through the skin, not lying on top. It glows with a peculiar, sickly pallor. It is jaundice.

'Right,' says the medical director, still at the central station, 'we have to think about jaundice, don't we?' He says it in a kindly enough fashion. He can feel the students' nerves. They are caught between wanting to impress him and not wanting to show themselves up. 'Let's think in pictures,' says the medical director, and begins to draw a cutaway diagram of the human chest and stomach on the back of an old pink form he has pulled out of a filing cabinet. 'Why is he jaundiced?'

'Is he pre-hepatic?' asks one of the boy students, flushing slightly as he answers. The medical director raises his eyebrows. They discuss hepatitis briefly then move over to the patient, who is now sitting on the edge of his bed, chatting to the large tattooed man in the next-door bed. The medical director smiles at the yellow man, who smiles back, looking up expectantly. He scratches at the plaster covering the drip connection in his arm. Young quizzes him on his history. It started with a pain.

'Where was it?'

'Across here,' he says, moving his hand across his sagging chest. 'But it's gone now.'

'And the jaundice?'

'I noticed the jaundice on Thursday.'

'And your motions?'

'They're a bit paler, and my urine is a bit darker . . .'

'And your general health?'

'Oh, sometimes I don't feel very well, Doctor.' He runs through a litany of past ailments, of fluctuations in weight.

Young asks him to unbutton his shirt and starts to feel around on the right side of his stomach, talking to the students while he does so, explaining what he is feeling for. 'Now,' he asks, 'is there anything to see, apart from a lot of tummy?'

The students look baffled. Young continues to feel, muttering to himself. 'What I can feel is a gall bladder, but I'm not sure, take a breath in for me, in, out.'

He frowns and turns to the students. 'So basically we have got a yellow man. We had better do some tests.' The yellow man eyes each of them in turn, uncertain how to read this descent into the third person.

Young runs through the options with the students. They talk of stones and drain tubes and operations. The yellow man is listening intently, obviously not sure what is for his ears and what isn't. Young turns to him: 'Is there anything you want to ask?'

'If it's a gallstone, do I have a general anaesthetic to take it out?'

'No,' says Young.

He ushers his medical students away for a discussion, pulling out his pink doodle paper again. 'OK, if he's got pale stools, that means he is not getting bile into the bowel. I can't feel his gall bladder, so that fits with there being a stone.' He describes to the students the various ways that different alternatives can be tested for and knocked out. 'There,' he says finally, 'we haven't spent a penny and we've got it down to . . .' More frantic doodling around the cartoon gut. The students frown cautiously. Behind them another patient is going through his own battle with nerves. He has just put on a hospital gown, prior to operation, and carefully seated himself on his bed so that his bare backside is covered. Then a nurse ushers him up, saying she has got to change the sheet first. He looks as if he is awaiting the gallows.

Young looks over his shoulder at the yellow man, now back in conversation with his tattooed neighbour. 'Amazing,' says the medical director, 'he looks just like that Mantegna picture. What is it? *The Duke of Urbino*?' The students look baffled. He turns back to them. 'Now, what are you going to read up if you get a chance this afternoon?'

'Hepatitis?' says the boy eagerly, flushing again at his own boldness.

'No, you are not,' says Young curtly. 'Obstructive jaundice.'

The medical director eats in the consultants' dining room, a long panelled chamber off Central Hall. Three other doctors, all in their fifties and looking sombre and dark-suited, are already seated at the single long table. Around them, dour paintings of the great and the good loom menacingly as they fill their plates at the serving trolley. Since the dining room has long been deemed an embarrassment by management, it is paid for out of private subscriptions by those who use it. That tends to be the older generation of consultants. The younger ones joke that when you walk in, it feels rather too much as if a Lodge meeting is in progress. And anyway the food, wheeled in from the hospital kitchens, is variable at the best of times. Young, who is not a Mason but feels he should keep in with his peers, is aware of the jokes. He chooses the curried beef and rice, and a banana.

No one really knows how much power the medical director has. Power in a hospital, even in a trust, tends to be diffuse. In a teaching hospital, it lies more often than not with the medical school, which controls many appointments through its panels of academics. But this hospital, muses Young, is not the kind of institution where people go around saying 'Oh my god, he's going to fire me' about anyone. The control of power is subtler than that, and fits well with the traditional hospital structure where all consultants are equally privileged, with equal pay and equal responsibility, regardless of age. Some, of course, are more equal than others, but it remains a fact of life that the medical director is as likely to be on call on a Sunday as a colleague 25 years his junior. 'Why do you guys have the same demands at 35 as at 60?' an Australian doctor asked him once. 'How come you don't shift into more administrative work as you get up the ladder?' Because generally, in Britain, you don't, Young explained. That is how doctors like it. It is strangely egalitarian, and not what outsiders – who hear lots about doctors' predilections for wealth and status – would expect. Although perhaps, this way, it leaves them more room for private practice.

There are those who bemoan the fact that hospital doctors have lost a lot of power but, Young concludes, that is probably power they didn't have much right to in the first place. Everything has changed so much, and patients in particular are not going to put up with patronising guff from an old chap with whiskers telling them not to worry, everything will be fine. He has seen how, in his own field of breast cancer, the whole approach has had to change. When he was a houseman he followed his surgeons, roses in their buttonholes and thumbs in their waistcoats, as they stood at the end of patients' beds and said, 'So sorry, you have got a problem with your breast but we will take it all off tomorrow and we're sure that will make it completely better.' End of conversation. For breast cancer patients it was, he concluded, a pretty shitty deal.

Now good doctors will sit at the bedside for half an hour, holding the patient's hand, telling her what is wrong, discussing the options, asking what she thinks. There is counselling and after-care, support networks and discussion groups. Most think it is the better approach. It might not be, he reasons, but the patients have changed just like the doctors have, they demand to be heard and there is no going back.

He got involved in doctor politics back in the eighties, forming a discussion group for young consultants called the 2000 Club. Hospitals have always bristled with such gatherings like a porcupine has quills, some prickly, some soft. Clubs for eating, clubs for philosophical discussion, clubs – so it is said – just for being a Mason. When the new ideas for involving doctors in management were floated, he was firmly anti. Then one evening he was persuaded by one of the general managers to draw up on a piece of paper how he imagined a hospital *should* be run. He did a drawing of 12 to 14 people, complete with titles and who was going to do what, and a vase of flowers in the middle. The manager said, that's how it's going to be: a clinical dean, six group clinical directors, then specialist directors below that. Marginally more doctors than managers on the Executive. One way or another he ended up director of surgery for three years.

Then the Tomlinson Report kicked everything in the air, the chief executive came in and asked him to co-chair the merger group with a colleague from Guy's, and that turned into the medical director job. Every trust writes up the medical director job in a different way. At Guy's and St Thomas', it is probably more of an advisory than an executive post, to one side of the medical hierarchy that sees 40-odd clinical directors reporting to six group clinical directors, who in turn report directly to the chief executive. In the managerial sense of getting doctors to deliver, the medical director is out of the chain. But in the organisation-wide decisions – decisions on future planning, strategy, job issues, public relations – it is the medical director's voice that counts.

So, like many hospital jobs, the medical director role can be as powerful or as ineffectual as the incumbent wishes to make it. Given that this incumbent does not wish to lose touch completely with his operating list, he is probably not as all-powerful as he could be. He has too much in his week already. It is divided, as every consultant's is, into eleven notional three-and-a-half-hour sessions, and he has opted to devote only two sessions to being medical director. Of course, he spends much more time on it than that. It just means he works 12-hour days. But as they whisper in the consultants' dining room, he *really* wanted the job. That's not what *he* told people – more that it was Buggins' turn – but hospital doctors are a jealous bunch. Stick your head above the parapet and most of your colleagues will shout, 'Should've been me!'

Then again, he does have an interest. Ask him to compare and contrast hospital power élites, and he can nod his head wisely, lean forward and give an eloquent discourse, replete with gentle irony and full of little digs at his less imaginative colleagues. In the old days, he would point out, hospitals were run by clinicians, whose traditional powerbase was the medical and surgical officers' committee. That then became the medical advisory committee, and in St Thomas' and Guy's case, it became the medical and dental advisory committee. Individuals controlled beds, but the clinicians' body would make policy. It wouldn't commission new ideas or new buildings, but it knew that its voice was the one listened to.

That was ten years ago and more. Now the hierarchy is more clear-cut, and involves a lot more non-clinicians. And, of course, power has shifted into the hands of the managerial classes. Some doctors have taken it badly. For a tribal élite which, with a lot of beating of drums and dancing round the fire, likes to choose its own leaders and make its own pronouncements, it is not a message it wants to hear. Likewise the change in junior doctors' hours. In the old days, junior doctors were owned by consultants. It was a simple system: you are my houseman, you will be my servant, you will sleep under the workbench, and in the morning I will come and kick you and we will go on a ward round together. It worked well in the same way it worked well for the medieval apprentice. The problem is that the swing the other way – guaranteeing that junior doctors should not work more than a maximum number of hours a week – means that no one has the time to follow anything through. Now the medical director suspects that his houseman rather regrets not seeing more of him. But it also means that a lot of doctors who were kicked around in their junior days find they have no one to return the compliment to. That, to some, feels like a loss of power.

No, real power is now wielded by committees and hence tempered with discussion and bureaucracy. Some committees, like the clinical advisory group, which tells the chief executive what the medical priorities should be, still have vestiges of power. This committee, which the medical director runs with the group clinical directors, can get things done. The problem is that different groups, such as the medical school or the hospital managers, have different priorities, and the hospital is just getting so big. And now they want to make it bigger still, to cope with the merger, and the ever-increasing number of patients. Oh, and they want it all done more efficiently. In other words, with less money. Tell that to the patients.

19

Andy has to come back once a month to see the consultant after his bike crash. He doesn't get any physiotherapy; the consultant wants to get his bones right first. Just endless X-rays. Andy wonders why he has to keep coming back. It's as if they just want to give him a pat on the back. Each time, he has to take his clothes off in one room. Put on a dressing gown. Then walk back across the public corridor in front of everyone to another room. Then down to the X-ray department and back. At the afternoon surgery they chalk up the number of patients attending that day. Sometimes it's as many as 64 or 65. Andy can never work out how someone can see 64 people in an afternoon.

He worries about all the X-rays he is having. He worries principally about his testicles. How many X-rays can you have before you become completely sterile? No one will give him a straight answer. Most times he is not offered a lead shield. He presumes that is because they need to see the whole pelvis. He asks them if it is a risk.

'Oh no,' they say, 'it should be all right.'

He still worries. But he gets better and better. And he has to go to the hospital less and less.

Looking back, he realises that the hospital seems to him to have a slightly organic quality, as if it isn't an organisation or a business at all, but a living, mutating thing. He can't imagine how anyone can run it.

20

The last doctor to run the hospital, the man who used to be chief executive before the Trust was formed, sits in a small modern office decorated with old furniture overlooking the front entrance of St Thomas'. He is a cardiologist and group clinical director, still high up in the hospital status structure, with a thick head of grey hair and the kind of cautious good humour that is usually found in politicians. He appears completely unperturbed at losing the reins of power – indeed, he professes himself to be an admiring adviser to the current chief executive – and is happy to provide his own narrative for the Trust's brief history. He says the merger of the two great old hospitals has, in parts, been botched.

'The real challenge was to get the message about merger across, and we've failed to do it so far. You have got doctors on the other site wandering round with Save Guy's stickers. On this site you've still got St Thomas' written on the building over there, not Guy's and St Thomas' Trust. They just don't want to do it. The chairman should have been out there three years ago shouting

"Guy's does not need to be saved. We are not closing the hospital. Thomas' moved from the Guy's site 130 years ago. It is perfectly coherent to put them back together. Stop shouting that you are going to be closed. Thomas' is just as threatened as you are by the merger. You are not being shut. You are being moved." But that hasn't happened.'

And it can be done. The NHS closed five hospitals, including St Stephen's and Westminster, both teaching hospitals, to create the new Chelsea & Westminster in west London's Fulham Road. A load of new primary-care initiatives were launched. People can see the improvements in services. Patients like the new hospital. The battle for hearts and minds has been won.

So how does he think St Thomas' will end up? 'I imagine eventually we will swallow up King's College Hospital as well, and in 10 years' time the Guy's site will be a university campus, perhaps with out-patients. In terms of health-care delivery, it must make economic sense to get as much as possible on this site.'

Which will mean Guy's loses nearly everything. And he beams the kind of beatific smile that says, of course, isn't it obvious? How can you possibly see a contradiction there?

21

Getting to Guy's Hospital from St Thomas' is simple in theory. A regular shuttle is laid on by the management to transport those who have commitments on both sites. The bus leaves every 20 minutes or so, usually packed to the gills with students who are expected to attend both hospitals. Young squeezes into the last seat at the back. He is accompanied by a journalist who he is taking to a meeting of the medical and dental advisory committee of Guy's and St Thomas'. He wants to show him what a medical talking shop is. He knows this will not be a popular move, as many of the consultants who attend the meeting, held every month, are still fighting the old war against merger. Anything connected with the medical director, a St Thomas' man, is fair game.

He is in an odd position. As medical director for the Trust, he holds sway over both sites, but of course as a St Thomas' doctor he is never completely at ease when at Guy's. There has been such intense hostility shown by many of the Guy's consultants to the merger that it is hard for him not to feel it is alien territory.

The bus drops them off behind London Bridge station at the back of the Guy's site, a maze of grim old streets and grimy Victorian buildings, many of which look peculiarly inappropriate for hospital use. To outsiders the site is always disorienting, appearing to merge seamlessly into roads around, without any sign of boundary or perimeter. Much of the main medical work takes place in a tall modern towerblock which jostles for airspace with the long grey offices built round the railway station. Administration is scattered into older buildings across the site. Young walks the journalist across to the Counting House offices, built around two venerable, elegant, cloistered courtyards, where the medical director keeps a room next to the chief executive's. His office is bland and impersonal, as suits a space barely used, with a couple of prints on the wall and some old wine and orange juice in a hospitality fridge hidden in a sideboard.

'Drink?'

'Not for me, thanks.'

Young opts for coffee. A young manager pops his head round the door. In the half-hour or so before the doctors' meeting they agree to go through his mail together while the journalist watches.

First item: a questionnaire from a manager on the NHS executive about the problems of being a medical director. *Do you think a meeting would be useful?* asks the accompanying letter. Young smiles. 'I always say no to anyone who asks if I think a meeting would be useful,' he says. It is the first law of fighting bureaucracy. But he ticks the box asking him if he feels he needs more management skills and knowledge. He knows these questionnaires are sent out with the best of intentions, but for him, all the NHS reforms have been a fudge. Either you create a proper internal market and things sort themselves out – which would probably be morally and certainly politically unacceptable – or you control the situation properly from outside, and prevent pointless competition that undermines patient care. Not some awkward halfway house where some GPs buy services and others don't. It is a mess.

Second up is a letter from a pharmaceutical company wanting another meeting to discuss the 'added-value services' it could provide for the Trust. It has sent the letter before and he replied: be more specific. It has just sent the same letter again, asking for a meeting. No. Someone else wants a meeting to discuss the cost pressures of the Calman Report. No. Someone else wants to check with him that so-and-so can go on another committee. Yes, certainly. And so it goes on.

The meeting is held in the lecture theatre at the top of the tall Guy's Tower. Around 40 middle-aged men and five women are spread around the steeply banked theatre seating. In front of them, on the stage, stand a lectern and a table. No one sits at the back, probably because of the jokes about the Guy's Tower overhang. The 30-floor tower juts slightly at the top, and the back seats of the auditorium run on to the overhang. Since cracks appeared in the concrete walls just where the overhang starts, both the doctors and the students who habitually use the theatre have been careful to sit away from the overhang. Nobody really believes it is going to drop off, but no one is taking any chances.

On stage, behind the table, a senior consultant in a three-piece suit chairs the meeting. The medical director sits near the front, waiting for his turn to speak. Behind him is the chief executive. Otherwise the doctors sit in little knots, occasionally whispering to each other but spending much of the time looking round to see who else is there and who is late. Most of the younger consultants rarely turn up.

The agenda for the evening includes reports from the chief executive, the medical director and the clinical dean, giving updates on building projects, new job grades, junior doctor dining facilities and the like. The debate is slow and methodical, with four or five regular contributors from the auditorium querying this and that. Two hours stretch ahead with the heaviness of a long, damp drive through muddy roads. The medical director is not a great fan of the medical and dental advisory committee, and those who know him well might even suspect that this evening he has brought the journalist along to liven things up. If so, he is not disappointed.

The chairman reads out apologies for absences, then welcomes new attenders. The last to be mentioned is the medical director's journalist, who is sitting at the back next to the Trust's head of public relations.

'I'm sorry,' says one of the doctors in the front row suddenly, 'but on that last matter, did you say there was a *journalist* here?'

'Yes,' says the chairman, looking down at a pile of paper on the desk in front of him. 'He was invited by the medical director.'

'Are you telling us that the medical director has deliberately brought a journalist in to listen to the deliberations of our private meeting? I'm afraid we cannot just wave this through, you know . . .'

Young, sitting by himself near the front, seems to smile quietly to himself. These kind of ambushes are fairly predictable. It is not as if anything they want to discuss is exactly controversial, but perhaps principle is at stake.

Later, Matthews, Young and a group of St Thomas' consultants cram into a lift taking them back down to the main entrance of the Guy's Tower. One of the consultants jokes: 'There would be a few smiling faces here if this lift cable snapped.' They all laugh.

But it is rather a grim laugh. They look at Matthews; for once he seems rather sombre, no longer the Cheshire cat in the tree, sitting on some secret or another. Maybe he's enjoying the joke. Or maybe he is miles away, thinking about his holiday home on the south Devon coast, near where he was brought up. Perhaps a nice cushy job running the local county hospital. A small hospital, where everyone knows each other, where the patients get real continuity of care, where the pressure and the politics and the poverty don't fray everyone's temper. With lots of time for strolling on the beach, and walking in the garden after rain. Nice thoughts.

If sometimes he feels *why do I bother?* you couldn't blame him. Why do any of them do it?

Money?

No, it is more than that.

The buzz. The profile. The people. The knotty complexities. The contribution you can make.

The cold air hits the men as they push through the doors on to the forecourt at the front of the tower. 'See you tomorrow then, Tony,' shouts one of the doctors, as Young and Matthews walk off towards the station.

WOULD GOD TRANSLATE ME
TO HIS THRONE

Those diseases that medicines do not cure are cured by the knife. Those that the knife does not cure are cured by fire. Those that fire does not cure must be considered incurable.

Hippocrates (460–377 BC)

'Books are worthless,' Abrenuncio said with good humour. 'Life has helped me cure the diseases that other doctors cause with their medicines.'

Gabriel Garcia Marquez, *Of Love and Other Demons*

1

The road that runs along the riverside edge of St Thomas' is long and narrow. Perched a few feet above the Albert Embankment, bounded on the river side by a tall stone balustrade, fringed by towering plane trees, it follows the frontage of the old South Wing, passing fire escapes and portakabins and chipped Victorian brickwork, along the side of the Shepherd's Hall restaurant and on to the North Wing, where it segues smoothly round the big white cube into the pebbled pedestrian walkways that face the front entrance. The road is used for deliveries and access, for sitting out and chatting, and for watching time pass. Benches and chairs dot its length. It has an unimpeded view of Parliament and the Thames and the London skyline.

A third of the way down, a short concrete ramp has been built along the balustrade, no more than three feet tall and six feet wide and bounded by its own wooden railings. Up on the ramp, in the shade of the trees and surrounded by pots of geraniums and Busy Lizzies, a straight-backed old man sits in a customised electric wheelchair. He is smartly dressed in slacks and sandals and an open-necked shirt. His grey hair is neatly brushed. At a distance you might spot a long white neck-scarf snaking down his chest. Go closer, and you will see it is a white ribbed plastic tube which disappears into a hole in his neck wrapped in a bandage. The tube is connected to a black box on a shelf at the back of his wheelchair. From the box comes the unmistakable phtt-pok of a small ventilator. Another tube, tiny and clear, emerges from his stomach and hangs loose under his shirt.

John was once an engineer in the RAF, and is old enough to have fought in the Second World War. As a Bomber Command officer, he patched up the planes and got them up in the air again, flying back to Germany. He saw London bombed and rebuilt, defiant. He saw half this hospital flattened in the Blitz. It seems a long time ago now. He is dying slowly with Motor Neurone Disease. His skin is sallow and drawn but his eyes are still sharp and his face good-looking. His hands, once his livelihood, rest immobile on the arms of the wheelchair, the fingers swollen and distended, the palms strangely shrunken. He can hardly raise his arms above shoulder height now. He can barely breathe for himself. He can only talk between gulps of air from the ventilator.

Each day, he says, brings a little less. Each day he sits on the road and asks why, in the name of progress, he is kept alive. He contemplates death and studies the sky, knowing there are no answers there. Only one answer remains: he is kept alive because medicine can. Medicine must do what it can.

2

Carole calls it the dungeon. She goes down there every day at two, sometimes snatching a bagel from the café first, eating quickly, without pleasure, filling a hole. Then down the steps, turn right, turn right again, and into Oncology. She sits in waiting room five, waiting. Three sides of chairs and no windows. June sits opposite. She has a lump in her neck and undoubtedly a secondary one somewhere else in the same area, as they are bombarding her head with enormous amounts of radiation. She cannot taste or swallow. There is another woman outside who cannot sit down. Carole wonders what kind of cancer that would be.

Her time comes soon. In the room with the machine she pulls off her top and lies on the table, naked to the waist, with her right arm outstretched in a lazy backstroke, like a bored bather waiting expectantly beneath an indifferent, man-made sun. The radiographer lines up the vast calibrated eye of the machine with the Indian-ink dots on her chest. Carole feigns nonchalance and looks at the masks in the cubby holes along one wall, little plastic shields with name strips for people having treatment on their faces. The sheer awfulness of it. She thinks of all the people she has seen down here, the young and old, with their yellow-greying faces, their headscarves and bandannas, their crutches and wheelchairs, looking so sick.

When all is ready the radiographer leaves the room. He speaks to her through a tannoy in the wall. She remembers the line from Solzhenitsyn's *Cancer Ward*. *You felt the door to your past had been slammed behind you, and the life here was so vile it frightened you more than the actual tumour.* It is how she feels.

Carole found her lump while on holiday abroad. She was on the beach, drying herself after a swim, when her towel fluffed over a little bump under her right arm. It was like a pellet, or a small ball bearing, spherical to the touch, dug in under layers of skin just to the left of her sweat glands. It wasn't sore or itchy, just there. A passive little intruder that seemed to have burrowed in overnight.

She didn't think much more of it. She was only 34, for God's sake, a mother with a two-year-old son and a 36-year-old husband. She felt great. Still, back in London, she showed it to her GP, who prodded it and says 'I don't think it is anything, let's wait a few weeks and see if it goes down.' When it didn't she was referred to the breast clinic at Guy's. She wasn't worried, just making sure, covering all the bases. At the clinic, another doctor prodded the lump and pummelled her breast, playing it like a piano with his fingers. 'No, nothing there,' he said. 'We can take it out if you want but there is not really much point.' No, said Carole, if you don't think there is much point, I don't either.

But her mother disagreed. She had had non-malignant lumps taken out when she was 45 and said that if they could come out, they should. Carole didn't know what to think, but her mum seemed so certain that, well, maybe she was right. She went back to the breast clinic and said she wanted it taken out as soon as possible. The doctor said, fine, we'll do it as day surgery next week, it takes half an hour. So Carole went in the next week, had the lump taken out under local anaesthetic by a nice registrar, who said, no, it doesn't look malignant to me, but we'll send it off for tests anyway. Carole went home and waited for the phone call giving her the all-clear.

Instead, she got a letter a week later asking her to come in again. She rang the clinic back and asked, can't you just tell me on the phone? You know, I have got my boy to look after, and it is a bit of a way in by public transport, and I don't want to waste any of your precious ... No, said the woman on the line. You *have* to come in. It is not our policy to talk to people about their results on the phone. OK, said Carole, if it's policy I'll come in. She didn't think there was anything wrong. All along she had been told it was fine, fine, fine. She was an optimist by nature. When her husband, who was not, said he would come along too with the boy, she thought nothing of it. It was near his work, after all.

She fixed up a time on a Wednesday afternoon. She got there early with her husband. Her son promptly fell asleep in his pushchair. When she was called in to see the consultant, she told her husband to stay put with the boy, as it wouldn't take long. She walked into the consultant's office and was suprised to find quite a crowd there already. As well as the consultant, there was a middle-aged woman who was introduced as a counsellor, and a male registrar she hadn't met before. She sat down. The consultant, who was young and dark, rubbed his hands together anxiously and cleared his throat.

'I am afraid we have some rather bad news for you,' he said.

Carole felt an icy finger run down her spine. 'I think I'd like my husband to come in, then,' she whispered. She hauled him in from the waiting room, wheeling the pushchair in front of him. The doctor then explained: the tumour was malignant, another operation was needed to remove some lymph nodes for testing, they would like her to come into the hospital in three days' time. He described the operation and then started talking about life expectancy and how, depending on what they found, it was possible that she might not be able to have any more children. She might have to have chemotherapy. By that stage Carole wasn't listening any more. Three days' time? She was too shocked to cry. She just looked at her beautiful boy asleep in his pushchair and felt so sorry for him. No brother, no sister. No mother. It seemed so stark. By the time the consultant had finished he had convinced her: she was going to die.

Afterwards the counsellor took her outside and ran through what they wanted her to do: come in the next day for a mammogram, then return on Sunday to prepare for the operation on Monday. But Carole was hardly listening, she was in a daze. It was as if she had just been thrust on to a rollercoaster and no one would let her off.

The next three days passed too quickly. Carole had the mammogram and felt they were piling indignity on indignity – first the mental torment, then the physical torture. She had to squish her breast on a plate and get it squashed out top and bottom and side. She hated it. Later she sat in a café for hours with a friend, talking over the possibilities. On the same friend's recommendation, she went to see a Tibetan doctor in Kensington, who gave her some vitamin pills and talked to her about what her body needed in preparation for the ordeal ahead. She visited health food shops and bought seaweed and other stuff she had never gone near before. She felt she was covering all options. That weekend she went with her husband to a wedding in Yorkshire. Her husband was distraught. While he got drunk, she spent the entire reception talking to a man who had just had a brain tumour removed. Later in the disco someone gave her an Ecstasy tablet. She thought: what the hell, I might as well take it, I'm probably going to die anyway. Then she spent all night fighting the effects, railing at her husband, worrying about how it would affect her operation on Monday. How could she have been so stupid!

The next day it didn't seem so important. The train down to London was late and she didn't get into the hospital till 11 p.m. She was second on the operating list. When she woke up after the operation at lunchtime, she felt fine. She had a bottle and line attached to her armpit collecting lymph fluid which she wheeled around with her. She did her photo albums and chatted to visitors, but generally avoided the other patients. She didn't want to share their problems, she didn't want to know what might be in store. The doctors said that she would get the results on Thursday, just sit tight. The waiting was vile, like watching your own blood run out, powerless to staunch the wound.

The counsellor came to see her on Wednesday evening and said she had good news, she had popped into the lab and seen her results, they were all clear. The consultant confirmed it the next day. Carole feigned relief, as if she didn't know – what she really knew, though, was that the ordeal, once started, is never over. The crab never lets go. 'You will still need radiotherapy, of course,' said the consultant, 'just in case there were a few cancerous cells left behind.' Carole's heart sank. She would need to attend St Thomas' for 42 days of treatment. The consultant tried to cheer her up. 'We reckon you have about a 93 per cent chance of surviving the next five years,' he said.

'Ninety-three per cent?' she queried.

'Well, there are buses,' he laughed.

It took her a second to get the joke.

3

There is a beauty as well as a brutality to surgery. The way things come apart and the way things are put together. The way the surgeon can take organs out and something else will just slot into its space. The way in which, if at first you don't find what you want, you can keep looking. You can rummage.

'This lady is in her forties and has a tumour in her pancreas which is making insulin. This causes problems with her blood sugar, which has made her feel giddy.' Tony Young, gloved hands already smeared with blood from the open wound, is addressing a video camera held four feet from the operating table. So rare is the operation he is conducting – he sees only about one or two cases a year – that he has asked a junior doctor from endocrinology to film it for teaching purposes. The camera, tripod and fumbled attempts at directing add a surreal air to the morning's procedures.

Young and his registrar stand either side of the patient, heads down, fingers busy. A pile of swabs sit to one side of the wound. Gowned and masked onlookers drift in and out of the theatre. The cameraman checks what he's filmed in the eyepiece. 'It's good,' he says, sounding rather surprised. 'No camera shake at all.'

'OK,' says Young. 'Now I will show you the pancreas.' The patient's insides are delicately eased out of her abdomen, purple and red skin-sacs shiny with blood and flecked with yellow fat. The transverse colon looks squidgy, like a water-filled balloon. The cameraman mounts a little metal pedestal next to the operating table. The camera is now directly above the patient's stomach. Young swabs the wound. 'Nothing worse than videos covered in blood,' he mutters. 'Right, I am going to move the colon back. Here is the pancreas, we have mobilised up the tail and in the tail is the tumour. It is quite firm . . . a definite tumour there . . .' His fingers are working what looks like a little knot of gristly, fatty flesh. Now he is talking more to himself than the camera as he works. 'We always tell young surgeons never to make a hole in the pancreas . . . there are quite a lot of blood vessels here which make life difficult . . . it also produces pancreatic juices which digest things – the problem is the juices can't tell the difference between other organs and lunch . . . Babcock, please.'

'Now you should film the anaesthetist too,' says Young, giving a little chuckle, 'the heckler from the cheap seats.' His anaesthetist, young and pale, gives a little start. He has been wrapped in concentration, studying his bank of machines behind the patient's head. Young explains his joke: a cardiac surgeon used the term to deride anaesthetists on television the week before. The anaesthetist, a sharp-tongued Welshman, grins beneath his theatre cap. 'That boyo will never work in London again, I tell you,' he says, growling with mock aggression. Then he smiles and chats to the cameraman. They agree there is really not much to film down his end, so he had better take his camera somewhere else.

The scrub nurse puts a large plastic tube into the abdomen to suck out the excess blood. Another young doctor has come in to watch. 'Here's the tumour,' says Young, extracting a little lump of gristle. It sits on the end of his finger like an albino slug. He slices it very carefully with his scalpel, a delicate, controlled run of the blade, just avoiding his finger. The tumour bends slowly open. He examines it closely, small oblong glasses perched at the end of his nose. 'Here we are,' he says, addressing the camera again. 'It's very well encapsulated, not quite as purple as . . .'

He talks for a minute, then pops the sliced tumour into a little plastic jar and sends one of the observers off with the specimen to be analysed. Now he is concentrating again on the abdomen, feeling around with his fingers, looking for something. Slowly the mood alters to one of studied concentration. The team senses something has changed. In the modern world, surgeons generally know what they are after when they operate. The problem has been diagnosed beforehand. But there can always be complications. Something is not where you expect it to be. Something else pops up. A good team can tell everything from the smallest wrinkle of the surgeon's brow.

More of the digestive system is coming out of the wound now. 'Look at this,' says Young, working with his assistant. 'It's a huge colon.' Their heads are almost touching over the patient. 'Will you scrub up?' says the medical director to another doctor, who is observing. 'We're going to need you.' They examine the appendix. 'It looks like a little bit of appendicitis,' says the surgeon, pointing out a hardening of the white, worm-like rod of flesh.

'Do we take it out?' asks the assistant.

'No,' says Young, 'because of the faeces . . . huge lymphatics too . . .'

He plunges his hand right into the abdomen up to the wrist, pulls out more organs, casually, as if they haven't been in working use for years. 'Wet cloth, please.' He's heading for the spleen. Already he is thinking he may have to remove it. You cannot take out the back end of the pancreas, where the tumour was, without taking out the spleen as well. Suddenly blood spills everywhere, splashing up on the green gowns of the surgeon and his assistant. It dries to a dark colourless stain as they work.

The spleen is smooth and crimson, as big as an Irishman's fist. The cameraman isn't sure whether to film or not. Young explains as he works: 'You set off to do one operation and now we are doing another. That can lead to problems . . .' It is nearly two hours since he started, and he is beginning to wonder just how difficult this might be. He allocated two and a half hours for the operation – he has a patient with a breast tumour to follow. Then a flight to Strasbourg in the afternoon.

'Remind me why you are going?' asks the anaesthetist.

'I'm going,' says Young, adding another bloody swab to the pile, 'in order to learn how to do these endoscopically.' In other words, without invasive surgery. In a hundred years, operations like this will seem as brutal as an 18th-century amputation. In a hundred years, medicine's capabilities may be boundless.

'OK, let's have some ties. Can you remove these swabs, please? Blood sugar?'

'Funny you should say that,' says the anaesthetist. 'I was just going to do another test.' If the tumour was an insulinoma, the blood sugar count will have changed. 'What time's your flight?' asks the anaesthetist.

There are now nine metal clips with scissor handles protruding from the abdomen. 'It's all coming along fine, don't you worry about it ...' The surgeon is working with cauterising pincers, his right foot on a pedal that controls the electrical charge. The camera is running again. 'What we have done now is remove the spleen ... I was unhappy that the remaining amount of the pancreas was sufficient to drain the tail, so I have taken out the tail of the pancreas the length of my thumb.'

He drops the spleen into a blue plastic dish. It lies by the tray of instruments, harpooned by three metal ties, a forlorn piece of offal. A nurse brings a plastic sweet-shop jar over, three-quarters full of Formulin. Then she decides she had better put plastic gloves on first. 'Will it fit?' asks another nurse. The round neck of the jar is smaller than the spleen. It depends how much give the organ has. One nurse lifts the spleen with a pair of tongs and allows the blood to drip off into the dish, the other holds the jar forward. The spleen is dropped delicately over the opening, and slithers with a plop and a little splash into the liquid below. Forty years grown, a reject.

Young is beginning to put everything back in the abdomen now, gently but not with exact precision. The digestive system sorts itself out in that way. He is sewing up inside, using a small hooked needle and biodegradable thread. He holds the needle with a clamp. Each time he dips in and pulls out again, his left hand comes up to hold the clamp as he flicks his fingers over, repositioning them for the next swoop. The rhythm of his work is only broken by the dull thud of leather on metal coming from the other side of the patient. The anaesthetist, who was busy writing up his notes, is now getting angry with one of his machines. He gives it a sharp kick.

'Someone has got to tell the Trust that we need some new bloody equipment!' he says, his voice rising.

Young shoots him a dark look. 'And where are we going to get the money for that?' he mutters, still working. 'What shall we do, sack all the anaesthetists and replace them with nurse practitioners?' His tone is teasing, but the anaesthetist is getting riled.

'Yeah, you do that, Tony, and then just wait till the first legal action comes in!'

Young lets it hang. The banter blows over. He is stitching up the outer wall of the abdomen now, the operation is nearly over. The original cut runs north to south. He explains to his assistants that normally, if patients have a bit of a tummy, he would cut west to east, and the scar would be hidden in the stomach rolls, but this patient is thin, and north to south is easier. It's cosmetic, really, but the kind of detail good surgeons pride themselves on.

Finally the scrub nurse starts peeling off the Opsite, the clear plastic covering that sheathes the abdomen during the operation. The patient is ready to return to the recovery ward. Young and his assistants start taking off their bloodstained operating bibs. He was right: around two and a half hours was spot on. When the nurses have prepared the patient, they return to the table and help lift her off on to a wheeled trolley bed. It takes six of them, three either side.

Young gathers his notes and then remembers something. 'Can you make sure she doesn't have any dextrose?'

'Who? The scrub nurse?' shouts back a registrar. Young shakes his head. They all laugh.

'Is the next patient ready?'

'No, she's not up here yet.'

'OK, let's go and get a quick coffee,' he says. He looks pensive, perhaps still mulling over the anaesthetist's outburst. In a few months, he is stepping down from the medical director post to concentrate on his clinical work again. That, he concludes, will be something of a relief.

4

The chief executive has his own problems. You cannot slip a hospital's organs out, rearrange them, slither them back in and expect everything just to sort itself out. Two old hospitals like Guy's and St Thomas' have always done things their own way. For many who work there, change is not acceptable. The hospitals' immune systems fight back.

Matthews, not an aggressive man, is careful which battles to join. He is a civil servant, trained to sidestep confrontation. Right at the start he reached an accommodation with the medical school: rather than unpicking how the teaching side worked – which would probably have cost more than any saving won – he said, let's agree there are a common set of purposes. The Trust has to deliver services, the school, which is part of London University, has to teach and draw in money for research. Let's see if we can cover all that, and not get too fussed about the lines drawn between them. With such an accommodation, the medical school has becomes a silent partner in change. It is trouble stored up for the future (one day someone will have to unpick who is paying for what), but it makes the present work. It is smart management. It allows both hospitals to run, despite the constant complaints of many who work there and the weeping sore of a campaign to 'Save Guy's' which battles doggedly to prevent change.

Matthews, because it is not in his nature, rarely gets angry. He has heard the theories that he should have knocked the 'Save Guy's' campaign – save it from what? – on the head right at the start. But it is a more complex problem than just announcing that the two hospitals were twinned before and that Guy's isn't being abolished. For every complex problem there is a simple but wrong answer, he sighs, when friends ask him. Anyway, the campaign is well managed and well supported by local politicians (even if the supporters seemed more likely to live in Bromley than Bermondsey). And the Guy's staff undoubtedly felt threatened. So instead of tackling the campaign head-on, Matthews settles on a strategy of wearing the opposition down, by just being remorseless about the issues: saying this is what we want to do, this is what we want to achieve, you can rant and rave all you like, but we are not going to take much notice of it. It is just another wall to run into. We'll get round it.

In private, Matthews argues that the real problem is London. The whole process of change in the health service was launched by the Conservative government with huge publicity, and then as soon as the difficult decisions had to be taken in London – how many hospitals, how many specialist centres – the politicians got cold feet. They began to say, well, we had better get this and this in place before we do anything. Then they imposed ideas like the Private Finance Initiative, under which hospitals had to find private cash to fund new buildings. Then an election loomed, which meant that everyone, including those with the private cash, waited to see if a new government emerged with different ideas. And so the system started coagulating, and that in turn exacerbated a situation already complicated by a lack of organisational logic that squeezed out any management initiative. The medical school, which operated between two sites, was told that it had to take on King's College too. The internal market began to bury managers under roomfuls of paperwork. Contracts with outlying areas brought patients in from hundreds of miles away for treatment they could get far nearer to home. No wonder there never seemed to be enough money to get anything done: to buy new equipment, to renovate, to make safe. Half the time the cash was being panic-spent, buying extra bed space to stop yet another winter crisis as emergencies flooded in and knocked out the operations that had already been planned. And so, despite everyone's best intentions, paralysis set in – nothing moved fast enough, nothing got done – and tempers frayed.

The chief executive and his team do their best, but to the staff who work with their decisions, they just seem like a bunch of amiable tortoises, pulling in their heads and refusing to hear the thumping on their shells.

Meanwhile, all those in the hospital have to work with the consequences of the system.

5

At night, when the chief executive and the medical director and all the consultants and managers have gone home, and Bob the Bed has packed away his clipboard and the nursing staff have been pared down to the barest minimum, the site nurse practitioner takes over. She commandeers Bob's notes and patrols from ward to ward, from North Wing to South Wing to East Wing to Lambeth Wing, checking where the empty beds are, checking which wards are understaffed and which patients are causing concern. She likes to look each ward team in the face, to see who is where and how they are coping. You can tell a lot from a face. As an experienced nurse with extra medical training, she knows how to sniff out trouble and anticipate problems. Every incomer, every difficulty, every emergency goes through her. While A&E is buzzing, she makes sure that the rest of the site is sleeping soundly. At night, the hospital is her empire.

*   *   *

Rachel is on the tenth floor of North Wing when the voice from switchboard cuts in on her bleeper. 'Fire alarm. Smoke on the twelfth floor in Mitchener Ward.' She knows it is serious. She has been to many false fire alarms in her time as night site practitioner – probably about four a week, she reckons. They are endemic in old hospitals. This one is different, though. Mitchener is empty, which means it is a prime smoking spot for patients desperate for a cigarette. It also means that if a discarded butt has started something, it might have been burning for hours before someone noticed. And when the switchboard cuts in directly on the bleeper, you know something is up.

When she reaches the lift lobby she can smell the smoke. She turns into Hillyer first. All the 12th-floor wards, made up of individual rooms for private patients, run in a ring round the outside of the building. They are connected via fireproof swing doors. She sees the smoke as soon as she is on the ward. It is seeping under the doors at the end and is plainly visible through the glass observation panels halfway up, dense and grey. The senior nurse in charge has already got the patient in the room nearest the door up and out. It takes Rachel only seconds to realise the gravity of the situation. 'Evacuate everyone,' she says quietly.

They clear the two wards either side of Mitchener into a third. The patients, bundled on to trolley beds and into wheelchairs, look gaunt and nervous. By now the first crew from the fire brigade are squelching past in their waterproofs. They take one look at Mitchener and call in reinforcements. Their controller, immediately identifiable by his white hat, takes Rachel to one side. He wants all the patients taken down to the lower floors. They can use the lifts.

But when they push through the doors into the lift lobby, the smoke is so thick they can hardly see. Rachel orders the nurses to soak towels in water, place some over the heads of the patients, and keep others in their hands. They can breathe through them if the smoke becomes too acrid. They take the patients down in groups, clutching their belongings, clustered tensely together in the lifts. For all the firemen's assurances, climbing into a lift at the top of a tall building in the middle of a fire is a deeply frightening experience. But everyone is evacuated safely. When the fire has been put out, Rachel takes a look at the damage. Mitchener is gutted and black. The fire doors between that and Hillyer only just held. The nurses think: we were so close to a major disaster that it doesn't bear thinking about.

When the nursing staff are debriefed later that week, it emerges that the fire was burning for two hours before anyone noticed. There are no smoke alarms on the 12th-floor wards. The nurses are furious. No smoke alarms? Why the hell not? Because, they are told, the North Wing was built before building regulations insisted on the installation of fully wired smoke alarm systems, and it would cost too much to put them in now. Some argue that the risk of fire now makes the rigorous no-smoking laws unworkable. Since all the smoking rooms were removed, patients and relatives simply hide in corners to have a quick puff. If management cannot enforce the no-smoking stipulation, they have to bring back proper places to smoke. Everyone agrees they will think about it.

There is a lot of grumbling but the staff carry on regardless. They have learnt not to rock the boat. Perhaps they have become immune to the risk of death too. It is part of their pattern of life, after all.

6

What is the truth? A hospital is an accident waiting to happen.

7

The woman in the isolation room is young, pretty and sick with the most virulent form of tuberculosis: multidrug-resistant TB. Most of the time she lies on her bed, coughing and wheezing, wired up to drip-feed and drain lines. There, up on the 10th floor of the hospital, she can soak up the sun through the large picture window, and gaze at the view of south London stretched beneath her. Occasionally she feels better and gets up and about. A visitor to one of the neighbouring patients watches her as she struggles down the adjacent ward, using her drip as a walking stick, stopping to cough every now and then. She must have been good-looking once, he thinks. African? West Indian? He can't tell. He wonders what is wrong with her.

8

Dr Alison Mitchell works in GUM. She is short, in her early forties, and wears a mousy bob with a puckish smile. She uses the smile a lot, to reassure, to grimace, to grin sardonically. You need a sense of humour to work in genito-urinary medicine: you see too much death and too many poxy private parts to keep a straight face all the time.

A fine grasp of acronyms helps too. GUM was the basement practice of medicine for most of the century, dealing with endless waves of sexually transmitted diseases (STDs) – 'Drop your trousers please, Mr Smith' – until AIDS came along. Now other consultants grumble that its out-patients department is the only one with carpet in it, and GUM doctors are getting too much publicity. But as a department it pulls in large sums of money for the hospital. Big cities like London have no shortage of interesting STDs to work on, not least among the growing HIV community. Within that, certain groups predominate: gay men, drug-users, immigrants. To STD specialists, who take a rational view of these things, there is just no point in working in the provinces. 'People don't have sex in the country, and if they do, they always have it with people they know very well and don't catch anything very much,' Mitchell tells those who ask. 'It's also hard to get a fix in the country and you can't be gay there, either.' In big cities, it is easier to find kindred spirits.

And St Thomas' has a track record with the HIV community. It was to St Thomas' that the 37-year-old Terrence Higgins went in 1982 with pneumonia and a depressed immune system. When he died in July of the same year he became Britain's first AIDS casualty, and had what was to become the country's best-known

AIDS charity named after him. Now Thomas' GUM unit has a budget of millions and light, airy offices in the Lambeth Wing. On heavy days at its walk-in STD clinic it will see over 200 men and women at any one session. There are special gay men's clinics, HIV clinics and women-only clinics. There are also rumours of big donations, new purpose-built premises, more staff and extra facilities to come. For the older doctors, the sort who lunch regularly in the consultants' dining room, the rise of GUM is rather perplexing. In their day, GUM was the sort of thing you only did if you couldn't do anything else.

Mitchell comes from a medical family. Her father was an ENT surgeon, she has cousins and uncles who were doctors too. Her father did not encourage her – quite the reverse, he tried to dissuade her, he thought all women doctors were hard. But eventually he relented, though he insisted she went to St Thomas' to train, not to his old hospital, St Mary's. 'You will probably marry a man from your medical school,' he said. 'Thomas' men are gentlemen and Mary's aren't.' She married a Mary's man anyway, and the marriage didn't last, so maybe her father was right.

The Thomas' she found in the early seventies still had all the trappings of a male order. Most of the chaps came from public school – grammar school entrants, mindful of Thomas' toff reputation, simply applied elsewhere. There was one Asian student and one white Zimbabwean in her year. A quarter of the students were female. Several of them cracked under the strain and left before qualifying. The authorities then reduced the female intake to 20 per cent on the grounds that girls couldn't cope.

The male values were endemic. It wasn't just that the female loos were miles away, it was the whole approach to teaching. Time and again, she found herself brushing up against the system. When doing biochemistry, the students had to take a drug and then fill a test tube with their own urine, in order to measure the drug's level. Mitchell was outraged. 'How can we fill these?'

she asked. 'Don't you realise we women just can't aim as well as you men. Give us some funnels, for God's sake.' Later, when they were learning about ECGs, the teacher would only demonstrate on the male students. 'Why just have the boys?' Mitchell asked, putting herself forward. The demonstrator relented, and then had difficulty getting the electrodes on round her bra. 'Why don't I take it off?' she said. 'Oh, no,' was the reply, 'I'm sure we can manage,' and he blushed to the roots of his hair. That's what big old hospitals were like. It was as if they had never seen a woman doctor before. The female nurses were even worse, and frequently made it clear to Mitchell that they just did not want to work for women. That was not why they had trained, and they made none of the allowances that they would have done for Mitchell's male colleagues. Mitchell, who had worked as a nursing auxiliary in the holidays before starting as a medical student, found that the hardest to take.

But she got through it all. She trained, took jobs outside St Thomas', married a man from Mary's and moved her career round his hospitals. She ended up back at St Thomas' doing GUM. She had just failed an interview for a job in Pathology when a friend told her to ring the GUM boss. 'He'll give you a job. He likes you.' That's how it worked. By the time she was a senior registrar she had been sent to Singapore and Pakistan, great places to study STDs. Soon she was back running HIV and colposcopy (named after the instrument which, when inserted into the vagina, holds the vaginal walls back to allow inspection of the cervix), and the department couldn't afford to lose her. So they created another consultant's post for her. She was very happy to take it.

9

Steve had known Mark for three years before he died. They had met at an art gallery. Steve was 33, tall, dark, the son of a West Country consultant. Mark was 31, curly-haired, sharp-featured and funny. He had moved south to join the gay scene and escape an intolerant working-class family. He was already diagnosed as HIV-positive and had been to the clinic at St Thomas' when they met.

Like some who educate themselves about AIDS, both had little time for what they called 'the HIV establishment': the doctors, the researchers, the drug companies and the media who banged on endlessly about the fatal virus's obliteration of your immune system, and then proselytised a never-ending supply of prophylactics with terrifying side-effects to help you out. To Mark and Steve, the medical establishment had no answers whatsoever. In the great religion of medicine, Mark and Steve were dissidents.

Mark first got ill in August when they returned from holiday in Samos in the Greek islands. His chest was tight and sore. He went to see his GP, who told him he was suffering from pollution, prescribed an antihistamine drug and suggested he get out of London. They left immediately for Ireland. Three days later he was admitted to the medical ward of an Irish hospital with stabbing pains in his chest. The consultant had no doubts about his diagnosis: Mark had PCP (pneumonia), but he was prepared to discuss the options around medication. They settled on primaquine and clindamycin as a therapy, combined with nebuliser steroids and dihydrocodeine tartrate, a strong painkiller known as DF118. There was no sputum test or bronchoscopy. The

161

X-ray said PCP, according to the consultant, and PCP was an AIDS-defining illness. Mark had HIV, so it all made sense, didn't it? Only the consultant's registrar seemed unconvinced. He grilled Steve endlessly about what kind of room they had had in Greece. Was it clean? Who else was there? Later Steve wondered what he had been getting at.

After three weeks, the hospital gave Mark the all-clear. He and Steve returned to London, but Mark was still unwell: the pain was searing, his sinuses were pouring, he had terrible diarrhoea, no one could explain what was going on. Later Steve decided that Mark's treatment in Ireland had just covered up most of the symptoms without getting to the root of the problem. A week later he took him into St Thomas'. He was told the PCP was back. Mark was asked to run up and down the stairs twice in order to assess his blood gases. They were lower than they should have been. Septrin was prescribed. Back at home, Mark took it for five days before he had to stop. He was feeling constantly sick and his diarrhoea had got worse. He rested for two weeks in bed, then returned to the hospital for another X-ray. The doctor listened to his chest and recommended he see the nutritionist to sort out his diarrhoea. He gave Mark a blood test and asked for three stool samples. Mark returned home to bed. Steve watched him deteriorate: his breathing got harder, he felt sick, he ran a high temperature and a violent rash consumed his legs, arms, trunk and face. A community nurse told Steve he must take Mark back to hospital. Then the story gets complicated.

Steve's version: a week and a half after their last visit to hospital, he has to wheel Mark in. He is severely ill and has developed a dreadful reaction to the drugs. He sees Dr Mitchell. She suggests that maybe the treatment is not working because of his immunity to the antibiotics. No one is too sure. Neither the blood test nor the stool samples show up any infection. A new X-ray shows that his PCP is getting better. 'How can it be getting better?' says Steve. 'He's worse than he has ever been and you are telling him the X-ray looks better?' And the doctors turn to him and say, well, you can't be too sure of X-rays when someone's got HIV. Later Steve tells friends that he thought all the doctors were just 'pissing in the dark'.

Steve sits around the waiting room while Mark is wheeled through yet more tests. He flicks some magazines and watches the people come and go at the various out-patient clinics. By the evening Mark has been admitted to a small four-bed bay on Alice Ward in the main North Wing. The chest specialists still say he has PCP. Steve isn't convinced, but what does he know? He thinks the registrar would understand. He is young, not yet battered down by the weight of medical conformity. He tries to talk to him, explain how he feels that it must be something other than PCP. After 10 minutes the registrar is looking at him as if he is mad. The doctor repeats very slowly and very firmly, as if speaking to a child: 'Mark has got PCP.'

You little fucker, thinks Steve. One, you haven't done a bronchoscopy, and two, you haven't done a sputum test. Don't tell me what Mark has got till you have tested him for these things. Do you understand me? Don't fuck with me. You have not done anything that suggests that the diagnosis of PCP is correct. Mark has been ill for six weeks, so don't talk to me about PCP till you have done a proper test. If Mark had asthma, what would you treat him with? Antibiotics and steroids. Basically that's all the treatment he got in Ireland. Don't you look at these things and want to listen to anyone who has been with these people for a while? I am an intelligent person and you are treating me like a fucking idiot . . .

Later Steve hears one consultant whispering to another that Mark is a 'difficult case'. What is it with hospitals? he wonders.

10

A man dies in a lift when his ventilator stops working. These things happen in a big hospital. Not long after, a patient asks a ward sister if it is safe to go in the lifts, what with all the people crammed in them, some with wounds and diseases, the risk of cross-infection, that kind of thing. She admits she can't really say, but if he is worried, take the stairs. The problem with the stairs, of course, is getting past all the people who are smoking on the landings.

11

Sometimes, just when you think you have got a disease licked, it out-thinks you. Tuberculosis, the greatest killer of all time, is one such disease. Estimated to have killed a thousand million people in the last two centuries alone, TB is as old as time and, on headcount alone, deadlier than any other disease known to man. It can gouge holes out of bones, deform spines, and gnaw away at organs. Death is lingering, the symptoms – emaciating fever and a racking cough which brings up bright red arterial blood – distinctive, the disease itself, although closely associated with poverty and malnutrition, quite undiscriminating. TB is spread in the tiny droplets expelled when a sufferer coughs. You just breathe it in. John Keats, D.H. Lawrence and George Orwell all succumbed to the tiny and virtually indestructible bacterium. But by the mid-20th century, man thought he had finally found a cure: a range of antibiotics which, if taken together in a rigorously observed course of treatment, proved an effective weapon against the spread of the germ. For a few decades, at least, everyone literally breathed more easily.

Then it came back. Ironically, it was the misuse of medical drugs which has created its new, more lethal mutation. Multidrug-resistant tuberculosis commonly develops among TB sufferers who fail to complete the prescribed six-month course of treatment. Partial exposure to the drugs mutates the bacteria, which grow into a new, more resilient strain. Like ordinary TB, it attacks the lungs and can be transmitted in droplets expelled by coughing. While no more infectious than ordinary TB, it is more difficult to diagnose and to cure. Unless caught early, it is nearly always lethal for those whose immune systems are compromised, whether through being HIV-positive, or through being on drug courses designed to suppress the immune system (such as transplant patients). In very immune-suppressed people, TB can also attack the intestines, liver, bones, brain and lymph nodes.

Outbreaks of MDR-TB have been identified in America, Italy, India, Thailand and southern Africa, where a TB epidemic has run hand-in-hand with a leap in HIV infection. Failure to monitor patients as they take their medication has led, in southern Africa, to the world's highest incidence of drug-resistant forms of the disease. Some doctors fear that the epidemic will swiftly spread north to the rest of Africa and the developed world.

Lucy was born in Africa but is now living in London. She is young and good-looking, but sick. She has been referred to St Thomas' by her GP. She has a one-month history of fevers and rigors, and a provisional diagnosis of malaria. A sputum test indicates she has tuberculosis. She is put on a ward in the East Wing and given rifampicin, isoniazid, pyrazinamide and ethambutol, a strong enough cocktail to wipe out conventional TB, provided she sticks to the course of treatment. Having been told what to do, she is discharged and given an out-patient's appointment for six weeks later.

When she returns, she complains of a persistent cough and night sweats. Her sputum still tests positive for mycobacteria tuberculosis. She insists she has been compliant with the treatment. She is put on a side ward for a week, given a final sputum test, then discharged on the same course of treatment. The results of the sputum test come in after she has left. They show resistance to two of the drugs. She now has drug-resistant TB.

The doctors try ringing her at home, they contact her GP, they write to her. It takes nearly a month before she turns up in out-patients. She says she feels better but she still has mycobacteria in her sputum. A month later she is back in hospital, in a side room off a ward in East Wing, suffering from fever and racking cough. A doctor suggests that she should be put on intravenous antituberculous therapy to ensure compliance, and asks for her movements and visits to be restricted to a bare minimum. It is also suggested that any health workers on her ward who might be immuno-suppressed be transferred.

A couple of months later, still sick, she is transferred to the North Wing, into a side room on Alice Ward, which has just reopened as the designated ward for thoracic medicine and includes among its patients many AIDS sufferers.

12

If you work in HIV, you get used to dealing with demanding patients. Every patient has his or her own concerns, and when their lives are threatened, they are entitled to be demanding. Being HIV-positive is never easy: it puts you in an intensely frightening, lonely situation. There is so much information to ingest, so many different viewpoints to listen to. Some patients just literally put their lives in the hands of their doctors, and say: help me, I will do whatever you think is best. Others quickly come to the opinion that doctors actually don't know much more than they do about HIV, and should realise that patients need choice. A good doctor will acknowledge that, and work through the choices with them. Such patients might be perceived as difficult by outsiders, but generally they are only demanding the sort of attention that anyone would want if they were sick. When patients say, I don't want to take your drugs, the side-effects are too awful, Mitchell does her best to persuade them that it is worth it, but she won't push it. There is no point in wasting a prescription if the patient doesn't believe in it. And if they query the long-term side-effects, she is blunt.

'The long-term side-effects, as I see it, are that you will survive longer,' she says. 'And do you really care what is going to happen to you in 20 years' time, when you wouldn't have been here in 20 years' time otherwise?'

But there are always some who stick firm, who resent being told what to do, who won't discuss anything, who question everything a doctor says and contemptuously abrade a doctor's self-confidence and composure. What can you do for them? Every so often one comes along. Mitchell describes them as heartsink patients, the ones who you swiftly realise do not want to be helped, and are looking for every opportunity to attack. The ones who when you see them you know that you are never going to win with them. She describes them as being in a form of denial. These patients don't want to admit they have AIDS. They habitually blame all their symptoms on the pills being prescribed to them, because that is their way of saying, I am not really ill. From their point of view, she can see that it is a thoroughly understandable way of dealing with it. They are petrified with fear and blame the medical establishment for not being able to help them in their predicament.

To the doctors who deal with chest and HIV problems, Mark

is swiftly becoming a heartsink patient. His partner is rude and aggressive; Mark himself isn't responding to treatment, and some of the doctors suspect he just isn't taking any of the drugs being prescribed. They are certain he has PCP, but his partner is adamant that he hasn't. In a situation like that there is little you can do but keep explaining quietly what treatment you think is suitable. But inevitably, more expert opinion is sought, which means more doctors, and Mark's partner getting increasingly agitated as his lover is passed from specialist to specialist. To him, it looks as if the doctors really don't know what they are doing. The atmosphere is becoming poisonous.

Mitchell gets that feeling you get with every heartsink patient: oh, God, I've got to go and see him, his friends and relatives will be there, they will want to know absolutely everything, and they'll disagree, he won't take the tablets, his condition will get worse, the doctors will get the blame and the whole thing will become acrimonious and fraught. But she does it with a smile, because that's her job.

13

Steve's version: he first notices Lucy when he is visiting Mark in Alice Ward. You look awful, he thinks as he passes her room for the first time. She is lying in bed, rigged up to a drip feed, her eyes seeming strangely enlarged in an emaciated face. He won't forget that expression. *Oh my God!* it says. *What is wrong with me? Why can't they find out what is wrong with me?* Sometimes he sees her wandering about the ward, slow and frail, stopping to cough. He wonders what she has got.

The doctors have put Mark on pentamidine for a week but he is getting no better. Steve is getting angrier. He's thinking, you have Mark on a gold-standard fucking drug for PCP and after a week nothing has happened. In fact his condition is getting worse, his skin is turning blue, he is not eating . . .

The doctors do more investigations. All they can find is an abnormal amount of the CMV virus, which commonly leads to pneumonia in immune-suppressed patients. There is no mycobacteria in his sputum. Mark is moved into his own room with his own toilet and treated for pneumocystis and CMV pneumonia. Steve determines to spend more time talking to doctors himself. The information he is getting is confused and bitty. Mark is becoming like a bewildered child.

One night he gets a phone call from Mark. He sounds badly distressed. When Steve goes in, Mark tells him that a surgeon has been to see him and told him he has appendicitis, but that he won't operate on him because he is HIV-positive. Steve says, of course you haven't got appendicitis. Well, says Mark, that's what he said. Steve waits for the ward round. A surgeon comes in. A female doctor who Steve doesn't recognise accompanies him. She stands by the head of the bed, head nodding, like a concerned policewoman. Steve sits in the corner, quietly watching. The surgeon starts prodding Mark's stomach. He goes, hmmm, hmmmm. Without saying anything, both doctors move to the door.

'Excuse me,' says Steve, 'before you go can you tell me what is going on, please, and tell your patient what is going on?'

'Who are you?'

'I'm his partner.'

'Oh.'

'I want to know where you get off telling him you would operate on him if he wasn't HIV. You can't say those things and then wander out. Do you have any idea of the effect it had on Mark? He was freaked out.'

The doctor apologises, and explains how difficult it is . . . Steve thinks he is waffling.

'I'm sorry, all I want to know is, do you think Mark has got appendicitis?'

'Well, in my opinion, Mark doesn't have appendicitis.'

'Thank you, that's all we need to know, goodbye,' says Steve waving his hand dismissively. And get the fuck out, he thinks, as the pair leave the room.

Another morning Steve takes in a friend to witness what is going on. In walks a GUM physician with 10 students to look at Mark. They all stand around the bed in their white coats with their hands neatly clasped behind their backs.

'Is this normal, so many people?' Steve asks Mark.

'Yes, most mornings,' says Mark.

'How do you feel about it?'

'I don't like it very much.'

'Well, you can ask them all to leave.'

Mark looks at the doctor. Steve says: 'Could you ask them all to leave, please? Mark doesn't feel comfortable.'

The doctor looks at Mark.

'Yes, I'd like them to leave,' says Mark.

There is a shuffling of feet and a few awkward looks, and finally the students traipse out. A registrar walks in and smirks as Mark says something. Mark loses his temper.

'Oh, get out! Get out!'

She leaves, but Mark breaks down anyway. 'I'm sick of being here, I just want to go home, I just want to be well. Get me out . . .'

The doctor sits beside him and tries to calm him down. Mark asks him about the PCP. When is he going to get rid of it?

'We never found PCP,' says the doctor.

Steve cannot believe it. He calls his friend over to listen.

'I'm sorry, can you tell us that again?'

No, says the doctor, we never found it, but we thought we should treat for it.

And Steve says, what the fuck are you playing at? These are

people who are immuno-compromised and you are prescribing drugs to them willy-nilly! It doesn't add up.

The doctor shrugs. Others say Mark has always had PCP. Getting doctors to agree is, it seems, quite a struggle.

Later, doctors say they have Mark in a separate room because they think he has MRSA. If he hasn't, he certainly has the next time he comes back in. He also has something worse. He has drug-resistant TB. The room they have been keeping Lucy in has faulty ventilation. Instead of taking the infected air out of the building, it is pumping it back on to the ward. There, a number of immuno-suppressed patients, placed in the ward to be treated for chest conditions, are being gently wafted with TB-infected air.

Steve's version: Mark returns to St Thomas' four months after being discharged. A red rash covers his face and his hair is falling out. He has been at home in a worsening condition. His temperature has soared to 40 degrees, he feels dizzy and has no appetite. The doctors tell him the signs are he still has PCP. He never took his Septrin. He is moved between side rooms in the East Wing and the North Wing. The doctors cannot pin down exactly what he has got. Initial sputum tests are negative. In normal immune systems there are just two mycobacteria which cause illness: mycobacterium tuberculosis and mycobacterium leprae (leprosy), but with HIV patients the choice multiplies. They treat Mark for MAI (mycobacterium avium intracellulare). He also has MRSA.

Steve is going frantic. He spends as much time with Mark as he can. Mark's condition fluctuates: occasionally he can get up and about, other times he cannot lift himself out of bed. He looks like a living corpse, wan and wasted. His room doesn't help: it is suffocatingly hot. He cannot sleep. At night, the patient in the room next door starts screaming, 'HELP ME! HELP ME!'

Steve has lost all faith in the hospital. He is horrified at the attitude of some of the older consultants. One in particular, he feels, cannot hide his revulsion for homosexuals. Steve watches him march into Mark's room and everything in his attitude says: you are a disgusting bastard for having caught this thing. You are despicable, revolting . . .

When Steve is not there Mark rings him up, crying, saying, 'They won't give me a bath, they won't give me a bath, please, please come in.' Steve says, of course. When he gets there he finds the room a shambles. Mark's pisspot has spilled all over the floor, his sheet has fallen into it, Mark himself is lying in his own excrement.

'I've had an accident,' says Mark plaintively.

'How long have you been like this?'

'A couple of hours, I don't know.'

'Why didn't you ring for the nurses?'

'They don't come any more when I ring.'

Steve puts him in the bath and goes to find the ward sister.

'This is fucking outrageous,' he shouts. 'Do you realise Mark was sitting in shit and his sheet was dipping in piss? What's going on?'

The sister faces him up and asks him if he realises how busy they are at the moment.

14

The GUM team don't know what Mark has got, the chest physicians don't know, the nursing staff are losing patience with his behaviour. When Mark is well enough he won't stay in his room, won't keep the door shut and won't wear a mask. He and Steve hang sheets over the internal air intake because they say the room is too hot. The nurses keep telling Mark: if they don't know what he has got, he might be infectious. To wander around like that is just irresponsible. He must observe the precautions. Then they find him in the ward kitchen, maskless. Steve too refuses to wear a mask on visits. Steve's attitude is: if you don't know what he has got how can you make us do all these things?

Then Steve goes in one day and finds Mark's room is empty. He thinks he must be in the bath, but then he notices all his things have gone. He asks the nurses: where is he? He has been transferred to another hospital, they say.

Mark's condition deteriorates. When Steve sees him next he is taken aback at the change. Mark is malnourished, jaundiced yellow because of the drugs he has been given, his backbone sticks through his back, his feet are swollen, his teeth suddenly look huge as the skin on his face shrinks away. He looks like a victim of Belsen. He dies three weeks later, of TB.

15

Steve's version: a month after that, he gets a call from Dr Mitchell.

'We are going to the press,' she says.

Steve doesn't understand. 'What do you mean, you are going to the press?'

'You know Mark died of TB?'

'Yes.'

'He might have caught it from one of the patients at the hospital. We are informing the press to trace other patients who may have come into contact with the bacteria.'

Steve is stunned. 'Oh,' he says, before regaining his composure. 'How nice of you to let me know.' He pauses. 'I don't envy you your job at all,' he says, and he puts the phone down gently.

16

The hospital launches a massive campaign to recall those who might have come into contact with the germ. Over 600 patients are seen. Seven cases are identified. An internal inquiry into how the outbreak occurred is also launched, under the supervision of the group clinical director of acute medicine and emergency services, who is based at Guy's. All the staff are interviewed. A report is produced. It concludes that the isolation rooms – which should have been run at positive pressure with clean air filtered in and old air ventilated outside the building – were faulty, the microbiology department did not enforce standard infection-control procedures, and that in future the chest physicians should not treat HIV patients on the same wards as TB patients (although it is standard practice at many hospitals). When the report is released, with the doctors' and patients' names removed, it is hard to see from reading it who is to blame for what.

They never name the victims. Who would benefit by that? The deaths feature in a television documentary about TB. Two consultants are interviewed and later regret their decision to let the cameras in. One HIV specialist says on film that if he had known there was an MDR-TB case on the ward, he would never have put his patients anywhere near her. Much of the footage is film of Matt Tee and the public-relations department handling calls after the announcement that 600 patients had to be recalled. Later a friend tells Tee that the programme made St Thomas' look like a big PR department with a nice little hospital attached.

With no names to chase, and a better story to follow at the

Chelsea & Westminster, where a survivor of a similar outbreak of MDR-TB is suing the hospital, the media move on. The Thomas' survivors keep a low profile. One, virtually confined to bed since the illness, is tracked down by a journalist. The former patient, already HIV-positive, contracted MDR-TB from a contact made on a day visit to the hospital. Just one day. He has a good job, which he thinks he might lose if he is identified. He is on the mend. He agrees to the journalist taping a short interview on the phone, providing he isn't named. On the tape his voice sounds strained and tired, but his tone is positive.

'Do you still have MDR-TB?' asks the journalist.

'I don't know,' says the man slowly. 'I'm still on treatment and still off work. They have given me a lot of tablets which make me very tired. I'm in bed now, actually. I've got to take all these tablets twice a day.'

'Did you know you had TB before the hospital told you?'

'No, they knew before I did. I had no idea at all. I just had bad chest pains and was coughing up a lot of sputum. I didn't know what it was. They told me and arranged for me to go into King's because they didn't have the facilities at St Thomas' for isolation and that.'

'Did you go into isolation?'

'I did. I was in for three weeks.'

'How was that?'

'It was terrible, really terrible. You feel so cut off, you just feel something is awfully wrong with you. You can't make contact with other people or be around other people. When people come to visit you they have to wear a mask and apron and gloves, disposable things.'

'So psychologically it is quite difficult to deal with?'

'Yes.'

'Did St Thomas' admit any responsibility for what happened to you? That you picked this up in the hospital?'

'They didn't seem to, really. I think they said they were sorry.'

'Are you cross about it now?'

'No, I'm not too bad about it now.'

'Have you been in touch with the solicitor who is handling the legal action brought by the survivor of the Chelsea & Westminster outbreak? I heard that some from St Thomas' were thinking of suing.'

'No, I haven't been in touch.'

'Would you take action?'

There is a pause. A faint, crackling hiss is heard on the line. 'No, I don't think so. I'm glad to be on the mend and rather thankful to be still alive.'

'Don't you harbour any bad feelings towards the hospital for what it did to you?'

'Not at all, no.'

'Do you have any memory of the patient who initially spread the disease?'

'No, I don't recall her.'

'Have you ceased contact with St Thomas'?'

'Yes, I'm now at another hospital.'

'Have they given you any indication as to how long it will take to cure you?'

'No. I've got to see someone again in a month's time. They might have the result of my last sputum test by then, and if everything is all right they will let me go back to work.'

'Are you still infectious?'

'No, I can't be because I'm allowed to go on buses and trains, and mix with people.'

'Were many restrictions put on you afterwards?'

'Yes, I wasn't allowed to go out much. I wasn't allowed on public transport or in supermarkets.'

'How are you feeling now?'

'I still feel tired. But I'm not too bad.'

The doctors get on with their lives. No one is blamed. The hospital did what it could. But there is always that wide gap between medical pragmatism and the indignation and disbelief of those who have suffered. No bridge will cross that gap. Steve sits in a flat in west London, appalled at the treatment his partner was given, his contempt for the great religion deepening by the day. He believes the hospital's initial insistence that his partner had PCP was motivated by money. He has been told that the hospital gets £75,000 for every patient with an AIDS-defining illness which it treats. No amount of explanation that this simply isn't so will convince him otherwise.

Alison Mitchell and the other doctors have to live with his contempt. For every angry patient and embittered, bereaved loved one, there are nineteen others who will work closely with them. Mitchell is struggling against a system too. She doesn't do the big doctor bit with patients. She always explains what she is doing and why, and always discusses treatment fully with her patients. She never gives drugs without the patient agreeing that that's what they want to take, and understanding what the side-effects are and why they need to take them. She fights for better conditions for HIV patients, and for young doctors, and for women doctors too.

She is the wrong target, but to outsiders everybody in a white coat looks the same. The circles of conflict spin round. The older consultants feel intimidated by her. They think she makes fun of them, calling them 'half-moonies' because of their preference for wearing half-moon spectacles. How dare she? they think. Sometimes you can't win. Everyone has their own version of the truth, and they are all right.

17

Up on his concrete ramp, John has a visitor. He tells him his story, gulping deeply between words. How he was perfectly fit till the age of 79, indeed he had never known illness, either in the RAF or later when he worked in the civil service. He lived happily in retirement near Esher with his wife; their three children had grown up and moved out. He had grandchildren. He was happy. Then suddenly he started getting attacks of breathlessness at night. His appetite diminished and he couldn't face food. He had no idea what he was suffering from. After all, nothing prepares you for old age.

The GP came to see him and asked him to take off his shirt. 'Look,' he said, pointing to his arm and chest, 'your skin is twitching all over.' He sent him to hospital in Kingston for tests. They sent him to another hospital in Wimbledon, but no one could agree on what he had. His back was getting weaker and soon he was having trouble with his bowels. His muscles just seemed to be wasting away. One consultant mentioned Motor Neurone Disease. Another consultant wasn't sure. Gamma globulin on an intravenous drip was suggested.

The next thing he knew he woke up in Intensive Care with a ventilator pipe down his throat. He thought he was going to choke. He hated it. What had happened? He couldn't talk. He could barely move. He felt the air being pushed into his lungs and panic roll over him. What was going on? He saw events through a miasma of confusion. It was like a hallucination. One minute he was breathing fine, the next thing he knew, he was flat out on a ventilator. He couldn't remember anything. His memory had been wiped clean as if he had suffered a bad concussion. He felt very frightened.

That was two years ago. Since then things had slowly slipped away. He loathed the ventilator pipe in his mouth so he agreed to a tracheostomy. He spent months in Intensive Care, first in Wimbledon, then in Kingston. Eventually he was assessed for a transfer to the Lane Fox unit in St Thomas', which provides specialised treatment for patients with chronic respiratory failure. He waited from November to May before the unit had room. All that time he was just parked in Intensive Care in Kingston, fed by nasal drip, waiting. He felt he was an embarrassment to the doctors there; they could do nothing for him. His only interest was in getting here.

When he got to Lane Fox a calm descended on him. For a time he felt as if he was living among the clouds. With its floor-to-ceiling windows opening out on to the riverside road, its airy ward spaces and sun-filled skylights newly built behind the old South Wing façade, the department seemed a world apart from the Intensive Care units where he had lived for so long. Most of the other patients were suffering from polio or muscular dystrophy. Many were out-patients who just came in for a week or so. There were always new faces and a jocular atmosphere. There was light and talk and laughter. The first few months were good. His MND was confirmed, treatment was prescribed, and for a time it worked, the disease went into remission. He got on well with the technicians, talking them through what he wanted on his wheelchair, discussing the possibilities, enjoying the companionship of engineers again. Then deterioration reasserted itself, punctuating his daily routine with a slow falling-away of capabilities. The doctors wanted to close his tracheostomy; they tried a swing bed to push his lungs into action; they tried positive pressure ventilation through a nose mask. None of it was successful.

John likes the people. Much of the time he is looked after by a male health assistant, a young Swede, who he trusts. But he has taken to brooding, sitting up on the ramp or lying on his bed. What kind of life is this? He is given temazepam to sleep. He has to have his lungs sucked out nearly every night. He cannot swallow. He has to have pills to dry up his saliva. He has to be fed through a tube. He has to be washed, dressed, pushed around, undressed. He fills his mornings by dozing fitfully, escaping reality, till noon. He spends the rest of the day reading technical journals and watching documentaries on television – he only wants hard facts, he cannot understand why people watch soaps and dramas. 'Why do people need fiction? Isn't life varied enough to keep their attention alive?' Then he goes to sleep again. Day in, day out. All he can be given is help to ease the symptoms. Nothing can be done for the condition. That, all too often, is the curse of modern medicine. To go so far, but not quite make it all the way. If he was a creature of nature, he tells his visitor, he would have been dispatched. He wishes he had never come round that time in Wimbledon. He wishes he had been allowed to die.

And he wishes that for the most practical of reasons. If he dies now, his wife, who he loves dearly, will be well provided for. He won't see his grandchildren grow up, he won't watch his children grow old themselves, but he doesn't want them to remember him like this. He likes the staff at the unit, everyone is kind to him, he is popular, but he has been there 15 months. He is incurable. He knows he has outstayed his welcome. There is talk of moving him to the Royal Star and Garter Home in Richmond, but his family would have to pay £427 a week for that, or maybe a nursing home in Claygate, but they don't usually take residents on ventilators, or maybe the Royal Hospital for Neuro Disability in Putney, if they have room. He cannot go home, because he now needs 24-hour nursing – that's three nurses working eight-hour shifts and replacements for weekends and holidays. He has worked it out at £50,000 a year or more. A rich man could go home and die. He is not rich enough. All he wants to do is go home and die, surrounded by his family. He went home at Christmas with a nurse from the unit. To have died then, oh, blessed relief. But it was not to be.

18

Only a magician can fix a head on a body, but any fool can lop it off.

Carole is deeply engrossed in her book. She reads *Cancer Ward* behind brown-paper covers sitting in the Oncology waiting room, devouring the words, avoiding conversations. She can sit like that for whole hours, only moving to sweep her black hair back behind one ear when it drops into her line of vision. The radiotherapy staff have started to tease her about the book. Carole shrugs. She just doesn't want the other patients to see.

She has come to feel resentful at the treatment, directing her anger at the great machine that she is convinced is rotting her bosom. She carries on because, she has been told, cancer can return at any time, maybe faster if you have had it when you are young. You have to do everything to hold it at bay. So she lies on the table each day, in the same position, breast up, arm right back. She feels nothing when she is lying there, the treatment is over in seconds, she hears just the barest click when it stops. But each night she notices that her breast gets redder and redder. After the first week she thinks it is going to fry, puffing up into a huge red bubble. But each morning it is always a little better, a bit paler and pinker. She writes in her diary: *Think I am moving around more cautiously. Don't fancy a bang on the boob right now.* Someone tells her that it might become rubbery and feel different, that it might be red for the rest of her life. Sometimes you don't know who to believe. She talks to the counsellor. They become friends, of a sort. By the end of her treatment she finds that only the counsellors provide the warmth and reassurance that you need. The doctors just won't allow themselves to get that close. Maybe they need the chilly distance to keep sane.

And already Carole knows that she will never feel the same about hospitals again. Her life was punctuated with hospital visits before: to have her wisdom teeth out at 15, to have her son at 32. But never like this, never surrounded by the dying and the very sick. And now she is one of them. To her, it seems such a sad place, and she feels desperately alone. Her life is measured out in windowless waiting rooms strewn with old magazines and hung with rack after rack of leaflets, and each leaflet she spots is about grief and bereavement. Death clogs the air and overflows from every sink and sofa. It follows her from the bus and stops in each café she visits; it cloys each mouthful of bagel and tugs at her elbow like a determined old beggar. It never listens to her entreaties every time she plays with her son. It never misses a trick. When she takes the long walk downstairs to the hospital basement, it's always beside her.

She doesn't want to die here, but these visits are gnawing the life out of her as effectively as the disease. For the first time she realises that a hospital may not just be a comma in life; it can be a full stop too.

19

Tee helps damp down the TB story. Rule number one in health PR: never forget the patients. The difference between a story with patient quotes and one without patient quotes is enormous. You can't tell patients not to speak to the media, but you can talk it through with them, whether they really want to, whether it is really in their best interests. It's a bit of a game: everyone gets dealt their hand and plays it differently.

Tee asks the survivors' doctors to talk to the patients. Do they really want to go on the record? Not surprisingly, they don't. News is something that happens and goes away. It goes away quicker if the patients don't speak.

Documentaries are a whole different kettle of fish. When Tee sees the TB documentary he is pretty angry. It shows the TV crew being manhandled away from areas where they are not supposed to be shooting, it gives the impression that the media storm is relentless and the hospital is organising a cover-up. But then his friend says 'big PR department with a nice little hospital attached' and Tee feels better about it. Sometimes, when you are inside looking out, you can get things out of proportion. The mess could have been worse.

Looking back, there are a number of things he would have done differently. Blocking access for the documentary crew was probably not an option, as they already had an interview with one of the hospital's TB specialists in the can. Tee suspects they had him saying things generally about MDR-TB which he wouldn't have said in quite the same way had he known St Thomas' would have to go public on its own outbreak. The first he hears about the interview is when the specialist rings him up and says he has already spoken to the documentary team involved, and sorry, he should have told him before. Yes, he should. In future, Tee thinks, he will be much more pro-active in sorting out with doctors in advance what they are going to say. He will coach them in what they might be asked and what the sensible answers would be. None of the doctors involved would have minded that, surely – they would have been grateful for the advice, because they just didn't know what the other doctors had said. They were being played off against each other. In fact, Tee thinks the documentary team were pretty sly in the way they went about it all, denying conversations with doctors which Tee knows they had, endlessly trying to portray everything in terms of conventional stereotypes: sniffy doctors, anguished patients, oleaginous PR people. Never trust a stereotype. The truth is always muddier than that.

But Tee knows they were only doing their job. It wasn't a bad documentary. After all, he thinks, it had people dying in it. And as for the stereotypes, well, the people who commission this stuff and the people who watch it like their stereotypes as much as anyone else. Put it down to experience. He knows now that he is better prepared for anything television can hurl against the hospital. Before the documentary team came in, he would have said to doctors: don't trust a film-maker further than you can throw him with a bag of bricks on his back. Midway through, he almost began to trust them – after all, they seemed a nice bunch of people. And at the end?

Looking back, his initial reaction was right.

20

A man, sitting at home, takes an overdose of antidepressants. Then he changes his mind and decides he doesn't want to die. So he rings the hospital and gets through to the sister in charge of the early shift in A&E.

'What should I do next?' he asks.

'You had better come in,' she sighs.

He is nearly middle-aged, tousled and unwashed. He sits in his jeans and V-necked jumper, grumpily flicking a magazine, waiting in the queue outside Major Treatment for over three hours. By the time the sister can see him, he is furious.

'You've kept me waiting so fucking long!'

She is stern but sympathetic. 'You don't have to use that language, please. Now remind me what you took.'

She returns to the central desk, where she wades through book after book, running her index finger down lists of unpronounceable names, trying to work out how toxic his drugs are. Soon he is pacing by her, his anger etched more deeply across his wide brow, hands thrust deep in his pockets as if tied there for his own protection. She picks up the phone and rings the psychiatric liaison nurse.

Later, another patient asks her how she can put up with that kind of behaviour.

'It's not for me to judge,' she says.

21

Everyone deals with the dead differently. In the hospital they live with the dead every day, they classify the dead, they examine them, stamp them and return them, to the fire or to the ground. So many have died here over so many years that each little tragedy appears to have simply thickened the institution's carapace, each little sadness just faintly falls into a snowdrift of cold consolation.

Strangely, for a palace of death, there seems to be little sense of God in the hospital. There is a chaplain, part-time, available for counselling, see the noticeboard in Central Hall near the statue of Queen Victoria. There is a fine 19th-century chapel upstairs, with seating for hundreds, nearly always empty and quiet. Occasionally it will fill for a memorial service for a doctor or nurse, an old-timer who gave half his or her life in service. But it is not an act of worship or faith that brings staff there, but of remembrance for a friend. They could hold their meeting anywhere. Most medical staff see no God in their world of suffering. Perhaps, as befits an institution serving a multicultural community, the hospital likes it that way. Yet to others it seems that their view is mechanistic and practical. Their everyday experience tells them that God is not there, and if he was, he might not be a God you would want to know.

God was there, of course, hundreds of years ago, when hospitals were run by the Church. God was there thousands of years ago, when holy men would trepan epileptics to let the demons out (some even survived). Now every doctor, every nurse, every assistant and technician does not need to attend to the worship of God, because maybe every doctor, every nurse, every assistant and technician *is* God every day in a hospital. They fulfil the role while God is away. *In loco dei.* God's locum, in other words.

22

Down in the North Wing basement are the big white rooms where all the bodies go. They are run by a short man with cropped hair and an irrepressible sense of humour. He has assisted at 14,000 post-mortems. He says he doesn't look at a cadaver as being a person. He looks at it as a mechanical object that has ceased to work, and his job is to find out why. Actually, what he says at first when you ask him is that it is a mechanical object that has 'ceased to be'. But mechanical objects still are, even if they don't work. Is a human being? Down in the basement, such semantics are rarely discussed.

23

Bill is first in as usual. It's nearly seven on a cold morning. He steps round the wall that screens the basement door from the car park and searches for his key. The morgue is a place with many entrances and few keys. Bill has one. The professor of pathology has one. All the doors are guarded by video entry-phones and strong locks. It's not to stop anyone getting out, ho ho, more to stop the unwary blundering in.

The lights are on and the sharp, sour stench of amine-based disinfectant immediately fills his nostrils, a smell he knows well after twenty years' experience. He has spent more time in morgues than out of them. This one, a state-of-the-art complex opened only a few years previously, is a quiet, soulless place. He steps around the corner from the car park entrance and into the morgue's main thoroughfare, a wide corridor barely 20 metres long. Down one side run two little offices, a viewing chapel and a waiting room with its own separate entrance at the back. Down the other run the fridges.

Bill studies the ledger. Busy night. Another six bodies have come in, two from the wards, four through A&E. Much more like this and they'll be full up, and have to start shifting bodies between hospitals. That means undertakers – you cannot ship cadavers around in ambulances, after all – and that costs money. And anything that costs money is going to make the managers anxious. And anything that makes the managers anxious eventually gives him grief.

In his office, second door on the right, he pops on the kettle and looks for yesterday's notes. The room is cramped and small, easily filled by three chairs, an ashtray, a noticeboard, a sink, a tiny fridge, a toaster, and a computer still half in its box. He lights the first cigarette of the day. He smokes non-stop, when he can. On the noticeboard is an old cartoon showing a woman standing by a grave. On the gravestone are the words SEE! IT WASN'T WIND AFTER ALL.

He sips his tea as he looks at the morning's work. Seven post-mortems, two different pathologists, both want early starts because of court appointments later; at least one of them – if past form is anything to go by – is unlikely to turn up till about eight hours after he's promised. Ho hum. He had better get everything ready anyway.

Out in the bright white corridor he walks down the bank of fridges, checking for the names on his list. Sixteen fridges, six racks in each, bodies slid in on top of the other like a bad night on a Continental sleeper. Doors at either end, opening into the corridor one way and into the post-mortem room the other. Each has a little white board with the names of its inhabitants listed in blue felt pen: 1. Smith. 2. Jones. 3. Evans. The fridge at the end has more names than most. That's where he keeps the babies and foetuses.

Bill sits and looks at his list again. He's tired. Getting up at five o'clock four mornings on the trot takes it out of you. He had one too many beers the night before last and is still suffering. No infected bodies, that's good, all the post-mortems can be done in the main room. He has to check on how many viewings there might be today as well. The bereavement officer will be in later. Then there are the bodies to be collected, hope to God there aren't too many going out first thing. On a busy morning, life is just one long rush from phone to fridge to slab. There is too much going on. Throw in a stroppy pathologist and your life really could be hell.

'So who's first, then, lads?' he says to the doors. The fridges hum back at him. He wanders off to put on his gear: a big pair of wellington boots, a waterproof overgown that stretches down to his ankles, a green plastic apron and gloves. He walks slowly into the cavernous, bright white post-mortem room. Everything is clean and quiet, just as he left it last night, the steel sinks clear of mess, the knives washed. Only the white boards above each autopsy station show evidence of yesterday's work, with their lists of organs to be studied: brain, heart, left lung, right lung, liver, spleen, left kidney, right kidney. There is a small pool of water on the floor to one side.

He squidges slowly down to the far wall, where another line of fridge doors waits for him – the flip side of the corridor fridges. He finds the door he wants and opens it: four cadavers inside. He pulls over a blue mechanical trolley. Pressing a small button he raises its height to five feet, then slides the second body out of the fridge on to the trolley on its steel bed. The body lies impassive, wrapped head to toe in a large white sheet, its feet sticking up proudly like the bow of a Viking ship. A faint stain, yellowy-purple, is visible at the head, where sheet meets steel.

Bill lowers the trolley to waist height and pushes it over to where the first autopsy will take place. The rattle from the trolley echoes round the room. He unwraps and removes the sheet. Inside is the body of a 69-year-old man, white, pale, virtually hairless, lying with his hands at his sides, a looked of stunned exhaustion on his face. He is two days dead. His skin is already papery. 'Morning!' says Bill, with a smile.

You don't grow up with a yen to be a morgue technician. Well, some people may do, but hopefully the system weeds them out. You drift into it. You need the work, or someone dares you. You find you have got the aptitude and temperament and you stay. Most cannot stomach it and believe there is something creepy about anyone who spends all their working life around dead bodies. But it is the meniality of the task too: no one calls a pathologist a creep. Technicians, who cut and display, who eviscerate and de-brain, who wash and stitch, who label and refrigerate, are the Igors, the Burke and Hares of the pathology process. But someone's got to do it.

Bill fell into it for a dare. He was 16, sitting in the sixth form at school in south London, flicking a newspaper, looking for jobs. He wasn't stupid, he'd got a knack for science and a bundle of O levels, and he wanted to work. *Job vacant, Sidcup Mortuary*, said the ad. Bill had a reputation for the sickest sense of humour in his class. 'Go on,' said his mates. So he did. His application arrived too late, but the mortuary at Sidcup said, don't worry, there's another job going at Guy's in Bermondsey. Guy's sent him an interview date. He turned up: there were three of them after one job. One candidate was two feet six with about as much meat on him as a butcher's pencil. The other was eight feet nine with knuckles the size of hambones. After individual interviews they were taken down to the mortuary to see who turned green. He didn't. The little lad didn't. The giant had a big smile on his face, which was quite off-putting. The boss, a bouncy little man who seemed, as Bill put it to his mates, full of life, chose him. Bill said, how much are you paying? The boss said, not a great deal but it's work. It was 1979, and jobs were scarce and about to get scarcer. Bill said, OK, I'll have it.

He thought his dad, who worked as a postman, might raise an eyebrow, but he didn't. He knew his son had always had a medical bent. Nearly all his O levels were science-based, but he didn't have the results to get into medical school. This was a step on the ladder. It wasn't even difficult work at first. The day Bill started, he was told he couldn't come in because they were doing a post-mortem. The boss didn't want to put him off on his first day, and sent him into the park with an apple and a can of pop. In the afternoon, he gave him a scrubbing brush and some scouring powder, and said, get started. And that was all he did at first, scrubbed and scrubbed, till his hands were raw. The mortuary was 200 years old, and looked as if it hadn't been decorated in as long. Filthy old tiled floors, rusty equipment. It all had to be cleaned while the place went about its normal business. Bill began to suspect the boss had shares in scouring powder.

One morning Bill came in and the boss said, 'We're about to

start a post-mortem, come and watch. If you feel sick you can go and sit in the park.' Bill watched, half in fascination, half in horror, as his first dead body was sliced up. The fascination won in the end. As the boss pulled out the dead man's organs, Bill even managed to name a few: heart, liver, kidney. The boss was impressed. He let Bill start by doing a bit of stitching up, putting the body back together again so it looked OK for the relatives. It is one of the most skilled parts of a technician's job. Bill took to it like a duck to water. When he asked why the pathologists didn't do their own sewing, his boss chuckled and said he wouldn't let that lot loose with a needle and thread.

So Bill did his training on the job, learning to cut, saw and sew, clip, wipe and swab, identify organs and tumours, and did it all so well that he sat his first technician's exam early, and passed with distinction. He flew through the diploma and by the age of 20 was the youngest senior technician in Britain. Soon after, his boss retired and he was running his own mortuary. When Guy's and Thomas' merged, he was running two. He was also pretty heavily involved in teaching and ran a lucrative sideline advising television companies who liked to get their mortuary scenes just right. The boom in detective series came at the right time for Bill. He was married, divorced and engaged again, and welcomed the extra cash.

He doesn't think what he does ever really affected any of his relationships. When he is having a drink with someone down the pub, he's always totally straight up about what he does. More often than not, people are fascinated by it and draw on his experience, getting him to explain what it means when their mum has a carcinoma, and why their uncle has jaundice. Bill is a walking medical textbook, remembering things that doctors never come near to finding out about. Working in a mortuary, he reckons, had got him more girlfriends than it has ever lost him.

And when people needle him, asking him if he wouldn't rather be a proper doctor than just a technician, he says, nah! Who needs the hassle? Down in the basement he's king of his own domain. The money's good, he can pull in up to £30,000 a year taking in fees for lecturing, teaching and criminal work as well. If he's short of a few bob, he can even go and do locum work at another morgue. Dealing with the dead is just a job like any other, and he's good at it.

24

A senior nurse tells her colleagues a story. Once when she was on nights they had a man who arrested very suddenly. He had only had a minor operation three days before, and then whoomp! A massive heart attack, no heartbeat, not breathing. He was 48 years old, it had been a gall bladder op, for God's sake, routine stuff. They tried for an hour to resuscitate him. It was no good. Later she looked around. Where was everyone? She found one nurse in the office sobbing uncontrollably, another in the treatment room crying. It upset her too, but at the end of the day he wasn't her brother or her father and she was a professional. She had to shake those nurses by the shoulder and say, 'Look! You've got 27 other patients who need your help. It's upsetting, but . . .' But what?

There was another time when she was wheeling a patient into Intensive Care and tears were streaming down her own face and she was thinking: I have got to stop this before I get there, I have got to stop this before I get there. She remembers her first few days on Intensive Care when she was younger. They had given her a baby to look after. She could hardly do it. Why me? Not a baby, please, not a baby. When she got home that night she told her flatmate, I can't do that again, I can't nurse babies, it's too upsetting, it's too difficult, it's not me.

When she got in the next day, the baby was dead. But don't say medical staff don't care. Don't say they are indifferent. Some care when they get home. Some care quietly in their own way behind their own defences. But when you are in the hospital you learn to screen your emotions. You make a barrier. Everyone hurts, but the patient must not see it. They judge their chances of survival on the faintest flicker of a frown. Everyone in a hospital must be an artful dissembler.

25

The ward sister sits at the main desk, surveying her patch like a contemplative cat, barely moving, controlling all with a cold flick of her eyes and the ruthless set of her head. Her demeanour has a purpose. There is a patient dying in a small room behind her. His wife is in there with him. The sister doesn't want anyone blundering in with tea or coffee, or doctors outside laughing loudly over case histories, or students giggling about their hangovers. The patient's condition has worsened; death will come any minute now. The sister has cleared everyone away. Her team know what's going on. They feel the change of atmosphere when she takes her position, cautiously immobile, feigning indifference. One by one they pass, glancing at the door, inclining their heads towards her, exchanging a look and a nod, and moving on, keeping the rest of the patients distracted, impervious to the slow eking out of life's last remnants just a couple of strides away.

One patient breaks through. 'I'll be in the day-room for the next couple of hours watching the cricket if you need me, Sister,' grins an old man in his dressing gown, paper under his arm, marching down the central corridor. England are winning. He is happy. 'Pure nectar!' he shouts. He has just been told he can go home that afternoon, his condition is not as bad as the hospital thought. There is a spring in his step. If only he knew ...

Slowly the nurses return to hover by the central station, all eyes on the door to the small isolation room. Suddenly it bursts open and a woman stumbles out. She looks crumpled and exhausted. The sister stands immediately. 'He's gone, Sister, he's gone!' says the woman, and then throws herself into the sister's arms with a despairing wail. The sister hugs her close, both arms round her tight, for a full half-minute. As the wail turns to sobs, the ward sister pulls the wife gently down the corridor, away from the other patients, to the relatives' room, out of earshot of the living.

Jackie steps out of the lift in a T-shirt and leggings. She is tall and broad, in her mid-30s, with a round face framed by bobbed black hair. She walks chin forward, head slightly back, a smile never far from her lips, as if looking for trouble, singing softly to herself, her rubber soles squeaking on the blue lino in time to the beat. The drive in from south London took nearly an hour this morning, and it still isn't 7.30 yet. She would have taken public transport, but since she got robbed last year – on the street, two youths, barely out of their teens – she doesn't like the walk home on dark nights.

She slips into the office she shares with the nursing manager and changes into her sister's uniform. Black tights, blue belt, flat shoes, name badge and the distinctive navy-blue dress with tiny white spots that is a St Thomas' trademark. In the old days, only nurses who qualified at the hospital – known as Nightingales after the nursing school's founder – were allowed to wear it, but that has changed now. In the old days, Thomas' nurses had their own reputation to burnish: 'Barts for tarts, Guy's for wives and Thomas' for *ladies*,' the Nightingales would proudly tell you. Jackie, like a lot of her fellow nurses, has little time for all that. She trained elsewhere in south London and moved on to St Thomas' when her hospital was closed. The influx of new blood, and the NHS's desire to create more homogeneity among the nursing profession, has done away with all the old Nightingale baggage, although the mystique lingers on.

It's a funny hospital, she thinks. Not as cliquey and old-fashioned as she had heard, and certainly friendlier than she had expected. When her department was amalgamated with its equivalent at St Thomas', she found the doctors courteous and charming. They came to her hospital, introduced themselves to all the staff who were moving, explained how the department worked at St Thomas'. She still had to sit an interview to get her job back, but that's life. She didn't get turned out on the street. It's odd though. When she went into nursing she never considered for even a moment that she might end up redundant. She thinks people always want nurses.

When she was younger she was going to be a teacher, like her parents, but she thinks now that she made the right choice. She works long hours – 13-hour shifts – but gets lots of time off. She's good at the job, and she has seen enough of life outside the health service to know that interesting work is hard to find. A stint serving in a pub when she was younger opened her eyes a bit. She didn't want a mundane life. Now, at 37, she is pretty pleased with what she has: a good ward, a tight team. The doctors like working with her. She is tough, opinionated, blunt to those who cross her, but fair. That's what you want from a ward sister. Every ward takes its character – its little rules and idiosyncrasies, its atmosphere, its sense of purpose – from the sister in charge. In these corridors, among these beds, she is the boss. It has always been so; all that has changed is the style.

In the first ward she ever worked on, an orthopaedic ward, it was frighteningly formal, which was how the sister in charge wanted it. Staff members were known by their surnames, all the patients had to be up and washed by nine, strict visiting hours were adhered to, no visiting was allowed on the day of operation. She just wanted to ask, why? She remembers little old dears who had come miles to see their husbands getting bawled out by the sister. No, you cannot see them, it is the consultant's round!

Please, you can see the sign, I don't care how far you have come, you must go away! In those days, patient power hadn't quite been invented. Now, of course, you are lucky if you can ever persuade a patient to have a bath at all.

Uniform on, she turns left out of the office and walks the 20 metres or so to the nurses' station at the centre of the ward. It sits on the top of a T, facing down a long corridor that runs back to the lifts. The ward proper runs along the two shorter corridors that form the top of the T, each with single rooms and four-bed bays off it. Men down one end, women down the other. Jackie doesn't think they like being mixed up, so she avoids it if she can. Twenty-eight beds in all, four permanently closed, run by six nursing staff, four trained and two untrained. All the beds are numbered, though there is no bed 13. There rarely is, in the hospital. Sometimes she wonders if the patient in bed 14 ever works it out.

She first worked on cardiac units at her last hospital. When she transferred to St Thomas', they told her they were building one of the best units in the country. Part of East Wing was being gutted in a £5m refurbishment to move all the cardiac specialisms on to one site. Her ward, halfway up the tower overlooking the South Wing and the River Thames, is a mix of emergency and elective beds, used for patients being tested for heart problems and those who just need what Jackie calls TLC – tender loving care. It can at times give her an odd mix to look after: mainly men, because they suffer more heart problems than women, middle-aged and older, some flaked out in bed, frightened and sadly flapping like fish on the floor, others buoyant and striding about, full of the vigour of Second Chance, on their way to full recovery. She likes to get them up and about as soon as possible. Mobilisation is part of the treatment. That is why she has banned televisions from the ward. Everyone has to go to the day-room. It is another of her little quirks.

But she is tough and cheery, as the job demands, and has a knack with people, changing her tone for each patient she deals with. She calls the lorry drivers and old dears 'darlin'', but treats the retired majors and bank managers with stiff deference. Everyone likes her, except those who have been bawled out by her. She has a fierce temper if anyone crosses her.

Only the week before she came out of the lift to find a man smoking outside the ward. She hates smoking. 'Put that out now,' she snapped.

The man glared back defiantly. 'You can't talk to me like that, and anyway, the sister said I *could* smoke here.'

'I AM THE SISTER, I DON'T LIKE IT AND YOU CAN PUT THAT OUT NOW!' she shouted. The man froze, Jackie's anger knocking him back like a punch on the nose. He dropped the cigarette and ground it out with his foot. You don't argue with a ward sister, not if you have an iota of common sense. Jackie brushed right past him with a contemptuous shoulder. Did he think she was a dickhead? Jackie asked her team later. She is not, by nature, a woman who likes to mince her words.

It takes half an hour to hand over from the night shift. Jackie writes notes on the condition of the patients, then studies the day sheet to see how many are leaving and how many coming in. The turnover is fast, like everywhere else in the hospital. As one of the cardiac centres of the south-east, they take a lot of patients in for tests from other hospitals. These then have to be taken back to the original hospitals for more care. Transport has to be sorted out, hospitals have to be rung to check they are expecting the arrivals, arrangements have to be made. The phone starts ringing at around 8 a.m. and never stops. Running a ward is not the kind of job where you can wander around mooning at the ceiling for long.

She sits in the staff room with the senior registrar and his team, running through patient care for the day. The doctors sprawl across the cheap plastic seats. The senior registrar is grey and urbane, smartly dressed in a charcoal flannel suit and expensive shirt, with a long stethoscope flopping on his tie. He looks almost a generation older than the rest. Two registrars sit to his right, slouching in creased shirts, one chubby and alert, the other dazed and suffering from a long, rough night. His short hair stands up in uneven clumps and his eyes look simultaneously tired and startled as he gulps coffee from a cracked mug. Opposite sit three house officers, younger, quieter, less confident, the pockets of their white coats distended by little books with titles like *Acute Medicine*. A fourth doctor, a good-looking young Greek on an exchange visit, sits in his crumpled coat in the corner, smiling earnestly, trying to understand what is going on.

The house officers say little. Jackie takes notes and answers questions when asked. The main dialogue is a prolonged banter between the registrars, who affect the sort of matey joviality which young doctors aspire to when performing before juniors.

'Do you think she should have some barium?'

'Well, I don't want to put her through something too monstrous.'

'A colonoscopy would be horrible.'

'All the patients hate barium enemas. Getting turned upside down with a tube up your bottom.'

'Like a Chinese torture.'

'Let's save it for someone else.'

'Like that nice patient of Dr Williams.'

'Yes, has he had one?'

'No.'

'What a nice man.'

'Shall we do a VQ scan?'

'Oh, I don't know. You know what they say when we do one: "If you think she has a pulmonary embolism, then she has. If you think she hasn't, she hasn't." It's a waste of time. You might as well take the money and go out to dinner.'

The senior registrar is enjoying himself, sitting back, arms crossed, his feet bent back round the legs of his chair. He jiggles slightly as he talks, a wry grin playing on his face.

The list of patients goes on. Occasionally Jackie butts in with an update. Mostly it is the registrars deciding who gets what. Sometimes they bring the house officers in with a question, just to stop them falling asleep. Would you give an angiogram in those circumstances? What do you think the liver problem means? What about the protein and albumin? The house officers sit up very straight and starched, hands dug deep in their book-stuffed pockets.

Finally they discuss the patient who is dying slowly in the isolation room behind the nurses' station. The tone changes, but almost imperceptibly.

'How is he doing?'

'He's OK for now,' says Jackie.

'I thought you thought it was RIP yesterday?'

Jackie shrugs.

The senior registrar shrugs. 'Well, he's had a very long ride round the River Styx. I guess he will be going soon.'

Everyone looks at their feet.

'What about the one we saw yesterday?'

'Oh, we've had to move him,' says Jackie. 'He wanted to talk nonstop and everyone in that bay was going crazy. The other patients were feeling rough and getting a bit angry.'

'How are we dealing with him?' asks the senior registrar.

'Not very well is the answer,' grins one of his juniors. 'His ankles are very swollen.'

The senior registrar beats a tattoo on his stethoscope with his fingers while he thinks.

'He did have some pain last night,' says one of his team.

'But he has had pain all his life,' says the senior registrar, still apparently deep in thought. Jackie sucks in her cheeks and smiles.

26

Down in the morgue, the phone rings. It is the first undertaker of the day, wanting to know the height and width of a body for pick-up. Bill says hang on, and finds the name on one of the fridge lists. He opens the door, slides the sheet-wrapped body partially out, measures roughly and walks back to the phone.

'Five feet six, little tubby one,' he says, cradling the phone on his shoulder while he taps out another cigarette. The undertakers like his relentless chirpiness. The blokes you meet in this kind of job either talk a lot or say nothing at all. Bill never stops.

He goes back into the post-mortem room, and sorts out which bodies he is going to get out first. The bright modernity of it all still takes some getting used to. The morgue has only just been to rebuilt. The last one was condemned by Health and Safety, leaving the hospital with no choice but to start again from scratch. For 18 months, while they rebuilt, the bodies were ferried across south London to Guy's for post-mortems. The only drawback with state-of-the-art facilities is that you don't get so many film crews renting the premises now. Too modern for them. If mortuaries really were as dim and Victorian as TV producers wanted, thinks Bill, they'd be pretty lethal places to work. He chuckles to himself at the very idea. He does a lot of chuckling.

He takes out four bodies in all, wheeling each to a workstation, and gets himself organised to work on number one. Most mornings he works with another technician, but she isn't in today. Then they take a body each – you never work together because of risk of injury from the sharp instruments – and the prep time is halved. But he is as happy working on his own, cutting and pulling so that everything is ready for the pathologist. Different post-mortems demand different things, but if it's your standard collapse, then it's organs out first, brain next, all ready for the pathologist to start poking around and confirming cause of death. The complicated ones are when they have died on the operating table and the surgeons have to come down and go through it piece by piece with the pathologist. They never need much of an invitation. Just a call: 'You know your patient that died the other day and is here for inquest? How would you like to pop round before you go in front of the coroner to explain what happened?' That generally gets them down pretty quick. Cancel all invitations, I'm on my way. Bill always laughs at that.

Not everyone gets a post-mortem, of course, but an awful lot do: coroners request it, relatives request it, doctors request it. They need to know, and the knowledge might help save someone else. And at least with a post-mortem, as Bill is fond of pointing out, you are more likely to get the cause of death right than just having a guess from looking at them. The last research he saw showed that over 60 per cent of death certificates get cause of death wrong. It may only be a technicality for the corpses concerned, but in medicine technicalities matter.

He reads his notes and then begins, gently running his knife down the first cadaver from the Adam's apple to the pubis. He removes the organs in blocks. He works fast, taking out first the heart and lungs, along with the blood vessels to the brain and the tongue. Next he removes the liver, spleen, pancreas and stomach. A standard evisceration will take him seven minutes, one with complications longer. The large room is quiet apart from the clang of metal on steel when he puts a tool down. He leaves the organs out for the pathologist to examine and moves on to the head. Steadying himself, he cuts from behind the ears across the head, through the hairline. Then he peels the scalp back both ways, revealing the skull. He saws round that, before inserting a T piece and twisting, parting a cap of bone from the skull and revealing the brain. He removes it, carefully.

It sits like two clenched hands in a dish, awaiting the pathologist. It has taken Bill twelve minutes in all.

He moves to the next body and the procedure repeats itself. When the pathologist arrives, he will find his body, have a quick check around to see that Bill has not missed anything, and take the organs he is interested in off to the dissecting bench, where his tools are already laid out waiting. If he's pushed for time, Bill will sit and take notes for him. If not, Bill will get on with the other bodies. When the pathologist has finished he signals to Bill, who bags up the organs, weighs them, cleans the cutting board and puts the organs back inside the body. He pads the neck and pelvis with cotton wool and then begins the meticulous process of stitching up and pulling tight, repairing the cadaver so that the post-mortem is barely noticeable. It's a skill that's older than the Egyptians. Bill works with cool poise, 400 stitches, rocking back and forth as his sewing arm works its way along the original incision. Then the head. Padding to stop leaks. Bandaging the skull back together – a nice touch, one of Bill's own, so the saw cut won't show through the skin – then pulling the scalp back over and sewing up, the stitches invisible in the hairline. Bill takes pride in his work. He reckons he's sewn up about 14,000 cadavers. Wash down the body. Disinfect it, redress it, put it back on the tray and back in the fridge.

The phone rings again. Its call punctuates his day. Usually it's undertakers or doctors fixing up who's coming when and who is going to be there. Then there is the door buzzer: three doors, always going, always someone wanting something. This time its the bereavement officer upstairs, wanting to send down a relative to view a body in the small laying-out room off the mortuary. Bill pads round to the office and studies the big ledger. It is quaintly Victorian in appearance, with columns for name, date in, removed by, list of valuables taken from body, undertaker's signature, age, sex, measurements. Everyone ends up as a statistic signed in and signed out, replete with paperwork, valuables listed, Free From Infection certificate, the lot. He checks the name against the book and then heads for a fridge. It has a large notice pinned above it: 'Please do not put bodies on top shelves if other spaces are available.'

He pulls out a body and wheels it down the short corridor to a door on the left. Through that is a viewing room, six feet by twelve, with a wooden headboard at one end. A window on the right looks on to a small waiting room. He wheels the trolley up to the headboard and gently unwraps the sheet from the dead man's head. He picks up a large red velvet cloth edged in gold braid from the floor and drapes it over the body and trolley, leaving just the head exposed. Then he props the man's head brusquely on a pillow, and wags a finger at him. 'Now, stay there.' Everything is still. The man's face seems sunken and drawn, frozen in mid-inhalation. On the headboard behind him a little basket of dried flowers looks mournfully on.

Bill goes back to his office. He never meets the relatives. Some technicians do, but it's not Bill's style. For his own sanity, he needs to be totally detached from the lives of the people he is handling. 'I am a scientist,' he says when asked why. 'This is what I do. It's the same as the people who work with viruses: they don't look at the suffering it causes but just try and understand how it works.' So the relatives go to the waiting room, view the body, and leave. Then Bill enters, removes the cloth, and wheels the body back to the fridge. It is his empire, but everything he does is unseen. He operates from behind a curtain of discretion. He likens himself to the Wizard of Oz.

The bell for the back door rings. It is a couple of undertakers come to remove Mrs Dickens. They are young, crop-haired and smiling.

'All right, Bill?'

'All right, boys.' Bill's accent drops into broad sarf London for the banter.

'Where is she then?'

'Over here. Got everything?'

'Think so.'

'There's your FFI. Sign here and she's all yours! Hang on, just make sure that's her. Check the number . . .'

'How's business?'

'Busy, you know.'

'Yeah, we know.'

Bill has never seen so many bodies come down as they have this winter. Either dead in the wards or in A&E, or brought in cold and signed off by doctors upstairs. It's the weather or the flu or something. Some weekends the fridges are close to being full up, and they can hold nearly 100. It's nothing to do with financial cuts or the merger or health-service reorganisation. Just a lot of people keeling over.

27

The curious thing about dying slowly, says John, is that as faculties are gradually withdrawn, memory becomes sharper. He can no longer eat or drink – he cannot swallow – and he was never a great one for gourmandising, but now he finds his memory of taste is enhanced immeasurably. He realises his memory of food and drink is far more pleasant than anything he ever ate. Savour it while you can, he advises.

What does he miss most? 'These,' he says, slowly lifting his ruddy hands off the armrest. 'My hands . . . were my livelihood.'

28

Back at the nurses' station, Jackie slips her fingers round her first cup of coffee and tries to get a sense of the atmosphere on the ward.

Calm.

Good. Behind her, in the two small isolation rooms, sheets hang over the glass panels in the doors, offering their occupants a semblance of privacy. Jackie would ask for blinds but she has no confidence she would get them. The ward is due to move in the next 12 months, and no one wants to spend any money on it. Lots of the little things are simply being left unfixed. But at least for the relatives of the man dying there, a sheet provides a bit of dignity. Jackie didn't expect him to last so long. He is a battler. But ward life must go on.

One of the patients, a wiry little old man with bow legs pushing out over his slippers, shuffles in from outside.

'Where have you been, Sid?' says Jackie.

Sid, a pint-sized 80-year-old Cockney whose blue pyjama bottoms flap round his skinny bow legs, is an inveterate smoker but always pretends not to be.

'Oh, just out for a little walk, Sister. Lovely morning!'

He lisps slightly. Most of his teeth are probably still in a glass by his bed. Jackie frowns. At least, she thinks, he isn't smoking in the ward lavatories. Sometimes the patients come out shrouded in fug. 'What have you been doing in there?' she asks them. 'Nothing, Sister,' they always say. And invariably they have got heart disease. It's enough to drive you mad.

'Should I give him this?' asks a nurse, holding out a drug bottle for Jackie to look at. 'Last time we gave it to him he dried up like an old prune.'

'No, hang on, I'll query it,' says Jackie. She has no compunction in getting the registrars to double-check their drug regimes. She has worked for over a decade with most of the drugs used on heart patients and knows them as well as anyone.

The registrars and house officers are congregating again down the corridor, waiting to set off on their morning rounds. One of the consultants has already been in, shortly after Jackie arrived, to see a patient who was worrying him. 'What's up, Doctor, couldn't sleep?' Jackie joked when she saw him. He smiled. In the old days the consultants came in at nine sharp, and patients could not even have a bedpan during their round. They just had to sit, washed and waiting, grateful for the attention. Now, with different patients in different wards, new work contracts, and shorter hours for junior doctors, you're lucky if you know when the consultants are coming, or whether the same registrars or house officers will be there when you want one. They are either in another part of the hospital entirely, or off on leave.

Most mornings, the consultants leave the mundane stuff to the registrars. They are happy to get the experience. They move from bed to drug trolley to notes, occasionally conferring in a huddle between the bays. Most of the patients are up, sitting in plastic armchairs by their beds, or chatting awkwardly by the large picture windows, looking out over the Thames and Big Ben. The mood is tense. Jackie always wonders how patients cope, at a time when they feel most insecure, when they are sick and think they are about to die, suddenly being thrust into a room to sleep with complete strangers, no privacy, people snoring, farting, sometimes dying on you. Most react in the same way, closing in, making cautious friendships, watching each other very carefully, looking for the slightest sign of decline, marking down each personal quirk. Right now, two of the patients are mulling over Sid.

'I asked him about those fags he always has in his top pocket. You know he goes and smokes on the stairs?'

The other man nods.

'I said to him, I said: "Is that your second fag or your first one?"'

The other man laughs.

'Do you know, he tries to tuck a bit of tissue over them and then says, "Nah, I haven't got any, 'onest!"'

'The only time he rings up his wife is when he runs out of smokes.'

'And did you hear him the other day, when his toast wasn't done enough, he said to the nurse, "What is that?" She said "Toast." He said, "If my old woman had given me that I would have given her the back of me hand!" Imagine that.'

'He's not looking as good as he was.'

'No, he's not, he was better before, wasn't he?'

Down the corridor, away from the chat, next to the posters about arteries and hearts that decorate the walls, the crumpled registrar is having his own conversation with the young Greek doctor.

'Well, of course, the best club round here is the Ministry of Sound, which is really famous now . . .' They stop to stare at a tall staff nurse, her bottle-blonde hair pulled back into a tight bun, lips like pale rosebuds, who smiles as she wheels the drug trolley past. There is always one. Both men seem to sigh a little.

29

If you think doctors have it easy, just think of what they have been through. Think what they have seen and then understand why they laugh and flirt so readily.

Imagine your first night qualified, out in A&E in a strange hospital where you never set foot when you were training. The real doctors have gone home. No consultants. No registrars. Just you and the nurses and the public and the white-bright strip lights which leave no hiding place.

'I remember my first night on call,' says Patricia. 'I was terrified. Suddenly people are expecting you to make decisions and no one is there to help you. The most experienced people around are SHO's, who don't know that much – after all, they were only house officers the year before. It was a long night, very busy, and this nurse came up to me and said, "We've got this child with a fractured leg, would you do me a really big favour and write up some pain relief, because his doctor has been called away to a trauma?" I said, yes, sure, and she said, just write him up some oral morphine, and I just went, OK, fine. So I looked at the child and wrote it up, even now I suppose I would do it.

'Then an hour later I heard someone stomping around shouting "WHOSE SIGNATURE IS THIS? WHOSE SIGNATURE IS THIS?" and it was the senior house officer and he came up to me and asked, "Is this your signature?" waving the paper in front of me and I just sort of crumbled and went, yes. And he shouted, "WHAT ARE YOU DOING GIVING THIS CHILD ORAL MORPHINE!" And I burst into tears, my mind went blank and I panicked, thinking, oh, God, what have I done, what have I done? He goes: "He's still in pain! You don't give oral morphine if someone has got a fracture, you give it intravenously!" Basically you give them a much stronger drug and I was so relieved I had given him too little rather than too much. I thought . . . well, I don't know what I thought. But it was the first time I realised that I was actually doing something that really affected people.

'The thing is, when you start off, most of it *is* bluffing, well, bluffing and relying on the nurses. They have been so good to me. It must just be hell for nurses, starting again every six months with a new bunch of idiots who know so much less than you do. And they were so nice to me that night, everyone gathered round and said it was all right, because I was crying, and that I shouldn't worry, and that just made me cry more! I'll never forget it.'

30

Bill misses lunch. In fact, he doesn't just miss it, he really yearns for it, but it's not worth going upstairs to the canteen. He's the only one in the morgue and somebody always rings, or is buzzing the doorbell by the time he gets back. On days like this, when he's on his own, he just sits tight and skips lunch. Smoke another cigarette. Same old thing. Everybody does it.

The pathologist who promised to turn up at eight still hasn't shown. Hasn't even rung. Bill has covered a couple of the bodies with wet cloths. You can only do that for so long, though, before the organs start drying up. He'll have to put the bodies away soon. The other pathologist who was due has been and gone, his mess cleared up. A third arrived out of nowhere, wanting to revisit a baby they had examined earlier in the week. The doctor was foreign, spoke bad English, and didn't seem to know how the system worked. He came back three times to get Bill to help him with the forms. Bill's mind is elsewhere, thinking about what to set up for the next day. Teaching day. Lots of medical students who have to attend a set number of post-mortems for their pathology exams. There is an observation deck that runs above the sinks down one side of the post-mortem room. It is bounded by a steel railing, under which clear Perspex guards are hung. They stop anything splashing up from the sinks – and, of course, catch anything splashing down from the students. Not all of them enjoy post-mortems.

Bill takes another walk round the room. He looks at one of the bodies. It is an old man. He has a small scar running down one cheek from his eye. It reminds Bill of the the old guy with the glass eye he had once. Been wounded in France in 1917, blind in one eye and deaf in one ear, in his 80s, died in a nursing home. He had a puckered scar round his eye socket. When Bill opened up his head and took out his brain he found what looked like a little calcified piece of bone, the size of a little finger, sticking out about three-quarters of an inch from a cavity. He thought it was a tumour at first, so he took a pair of bone nips to it and cut it off. It was an armour-piercing bullet.

Military gear is one of Bill's hobbies. He sorted out what it was after a bit of research. In the First World War the Germans had developed armour-piercing bullets to counter the first British tanks. The bullets were lead-coated, with a metal core, designed to penetrate 10mm armour plate and fired from bolt-action rifles. They were also used by snipers. The old guy was unlucky enough to catch one right at the end of its trajectory. The lead had been pushed back, it must have travelled for several miles before hitting him in the face, penetrating his brain, and then just stopping. It should have killed him outright. Instead it crippled him, and he carried it around in his head for another 70-odd years. Finally, tired of hiding, the bullet popped out on to a post-mortem table in south London. No one had known it was there. Now it stands on Bill's mantelpiece. He likes mementos.

Sometimes you find the strangest things. Not just shrapnel but spoons and nails. Then there are the S&M freaks. One corpse had a rope round his neck, pins through his penis, crocodile clips on his scrotum attached to a car battery. The ambulance driver who collected him said the battery was still live. You can't take the stuff off as it's evidence for the coroner. It wouldn't be the first murder to have been dressed up to look like an S&M accident. Murder makes it all more complicated. Head and hands have to be wrapped in plastic for trace evidence. Full front and back photos, fingernail scrapings, penile swabs, high-angle swabs, low-angle swabs, mouth swabs, nose swabs, ear swabs, skin pick-up for trace evidence, photo of each individual wound, measurement of each individual wound. If there are marks on the head you have to shave it and photograph it too. People always think that murder must be the most exciting part of Bill's job, but the truth is he finds a lot of it utterly boring. It is just procedure.

Like dealing with the babies. Some pathologists won't do them – everyone has their vulnerabilities. Bill, well, he reasons that he has to. 'I'm not in a position to be upset,' he says with a shrug to those who ask. No one likes it, but they get a lot at the Trust, especially at Guy's. If there is something wrong with a pregnancy, say a genetic abnormality, and parents opt for an abortion, then pathologists will normally carry out a post-mortem on the foetus to check on the genetic structure of the child. That way they can tell the mother what the chances are of it happening again. Then Bill boxes the foetuses up. In the bad old days they would have been incinerated as medical waste. Now they are handed over to undertakers, who take them to the council for a notional fee. The council donate crematoria time and burial plots free of charge.

It is not publicised much but it is done as a simple act of human decency. The babies who are never even born are buried all around London. You can find out where if you have the right number. Bill labels each box with a number. Any parent can come back at any time and find out where their baby went. Bill is, above all, a compassionate man.

So what does he dream of at night? What current picks his bones as he lies there? It's impossible to say. He just gets on with his job, and enjoys a drink or two in the evening when everything is locked up for the night. He never lies when people ask him what he does, and is always ready to dispense medical advice. He always tells the truth, however hard it is to take, because he doesn't see any reason to be untruthful. He sees the future clearly, without ruminating on what's gone before.

31

The problem with being a ward sister is where you go from there. Into nursing management? Teaching? There are grades and degree courses and other diversions, but basically it is a steep pyramid, with fewer spaces on each level. Anyway, good ward sisters like being on their wards, not sitting in an office. Like being in A&E, or operating, it is the buzz that keeps you going, the variety, the excitement of the unexpected. Some ward sisters leave, come back, leave, and come back again, loving the job, working on, right into their 50s. They just miss the teamwork and the problems and the patients and the responsibilities. But of course, being a ward sister is virtually being a manager anyway. The nurses do most of the hands-on work with patients. The sisters simply make sure everything is done right: the right doctors to see the right patients, the right patients in the right beds, the right beds with the right sheets and the right bedpans cleaned in the right sluice and the right drugs in the right mouths and the right treatment given by the right nurses. That's hands-on management. That's management by walking around. Who wants just to push paper? Ward sisters get to do enough of that anyway.

Jackie studies the duty rosters for the next month. She has been distracted from the ward round by the phone. She has a long 'bank' form in front of her. She has to tell the nursing managers how many holes she needs to fill in the next fortnight. The hospital runs its own bank of part-time nurses who it slots into temporary vacancies when staff are away on holiday or study leave. Jackie hates doing this kind of stuff, and is always late putting her forms in, but it has to be done. The problem is the distractions. Either the phone is going or a doctor is asking her something or a new patient has arrived. Just as she has got her mind round who is going to be there next week and who isn't, her concentration is broken by a low voice.

'Excuse me, Sister, am I in the right place?'

A large middle-aged man, clutching an overnight bag and flanked by his wife and grown-up son, has appeared at her desk. He has managed to dodge the ward receptionist further down the corridor. Jackie smiles and takes his name and asks him to wait in the day room, his bed will be ready soon. As the family wander down the corridor to wait, Jackie's eyes follow them, and her jaw drops incredulously. The son, dressed in jeans and T-shirt and with long, lank hair pushed back, has got an electric guitar slung over his shoulder. 'My God,' she mutters, shaking her head, 'I hope he doesn't think he is playing that in here.' A staff nurse glances over and giggles.

Jackie goes back to the ward round. The chubby registrar, who is just pulling the curtains round the bed, has to break the news to a patient that they will need to do more tests on his heart. The registrar has got a good manner, sturdy and decisive. His tone is just up-beat enough to lighten the message. Jackie has warned him that the patient, a taxi driver, is depressed. The heart attack that took him into hospital has jeopardised his job and sitting on the edge of his bed, looking balefully up, the man already bears the look of a fighter who is beginning to dread the bell for the final round.

'Now, we have got the results from the test you did yesterday,' says the registrar, making a show of flicking through the notes. 'You did a reasonable amount of exercise but when you stopped on the treadmill there were some things which suggested there might be trouble in other arteries. It's not surprising really. I think we should test them before you go home. There is a test called a coronary angiogram where we can take pictures of your heart . . .'

The man is looking at his hands in his own lap. A voice inside his head is screaming, 'Get me out of here now! NOW!' but he shows little reaction.

'My advice to you,' continues the registrar, 'would be to stay the weekend and we can test you on Monday . . .'

'I want to go home.'

'Well, I would let you go home the next day so long as we saw nothing awful on the test. It would enable us to decide on the right course of drugs or a better course of treatment . . .'

'I want to go home.'

The registrar adopts a sympathetic-but-firm face. There is a long pause while the patient contemplates his hands again.

'I suppose,' says the patient, 'at least I will be able to watch the cricket.' He looks disconsolate.

The registrar smiles. Jackie smiles. She begins to pull back the curtains from around the bed. They snag as she draws them. Half the hooks are hanging loose from the runners. She had an argument about the bed curtains with the linen department last week. Can you come and fix them? she asked. No, they said, we will send you some new curtains and you can put them up yourself. I'm not bloody doing it myself, she shouted, I've got better things to do! WELL, WE HAVEN'T GOT TIME EITHER! they shouted back. Oh, God, she wonders sometimes why she bothers. She loathes the linen department, they typify everything that is wrong with big hospitals.

Another man arrives carrying an overnight bag. Another new patient.

'Did you go to Admissions?' Jackie asks with a tight grin, knowing the answer before he opens his mouth.

'No, Sister, I came straight here,' says the patient.

'OK, hang on a bit,' says Jackie. 'Why don't you wait round there?' pointing him towards the day-room. She will have to square it with Admissions, and then check which bed to put him in and where to put the current occupant. Quite a few of the patients are leaving this morning, but she has to make sure they have all got transport. Some are already sitting in the chairs by their beds, packed and dressed, looking slightly lost, like wartime kids waiting for evacuation. Jackie has to juggle those going out and those coming in. That's what she uses the day-room for. It is like a transit camp.

Just then Bob the Bed turns up. He looks lean and well groomed in sports jacket and slacks, almost too neat for an institution where hurried dishevelment is virtually a dress code. His hands clutch the paperwork that is his constant companion. His face breaks into a grin when he sees Jackie. Their respect is mutual, two cogs in a machine who are not afraid to grind the gears a little if they think it worthwhile. Most of the nurses like Bob a lot – he is one of them. He has seen it all as a male nurse and he has a reputation for standing up to doctors who try to twist the system.

They go through his list standing huddled together in the corridor. Who's coming in. Who's going out. What's available. Bob jokes that one day 'the management' will find a computer to replace him, but for now nothing works better than pounding the wards, looking staff in the face. And Jackie for one doesn't fancy spending her mornings inputting the data that would make such a computer system work. That's not what she was trained for.

At her desk the phone rings continually, calls for doctors, calls for managers, calls for anyone passing through. The patients have their own public phone which Jackie leaves them to sort out. Where's Mr Wallace? a patient will say. There's a call here for him. Down there, last bed on the left. OK? When her own phone is not in use, Jackie is on it, calling out, organising transport for one of the men leaving, or a bed at another hospital that has to have a patient back after a check-up. Juggling beds becomes an art-form – sometimes she has one patient in the day-room waiting to come in, another waiting to go home and a third in the bed that one has just left. It's ludicrous or efficient, depending on your point of view.

'Can I have the bed manager, please?' she asks.

Eventually she is put through. 'I've got a Mr Dawes coming

back to you today. I just wanted to check you were expecting him . . .'

Jackie's face sets into a stony mask as the manager on the other end of the line huffs and puffs and then announces that no, it's not in his books, and sorry, they have no beds free at the moment. Dear God, she says, give her Bob any day. Where do they find these people?

'Well, I'm sorry,' says Jackie, 'this patient is booked to return to you today and if you don't accept him we will simply put him through Casualty.' When hospitals try to delay having their patients back, St Thomas' simply returns them to their A&E department. That way it is their responsibility, and the bed at St Thomas' is free for the next patient. It is a cynical tactic, but it works.

Next Jackie rings the ward the man is supposed to return to. Sometimes, speaking to the ward sister is an easier way of doing things.

'You *have* a got a bed for him? Well, your bed manager insists that you haven't, so you should tell him. That's great. We'll send the patient over at lunchtime. Many thanks.'

By the time she has put the phone down, a tense-looking young woman wearing a doctor's white coat and clutching a small bag is standing over her. 'Yes?' says Jackie.

'I'm the chiropodist, for Mr Forbes?' says the woman tentatively.

'But your colleague came in for Mr Forbes two days ago.'

The young woman's face crinkles into a frown. 'God, typical, isn't it? Thing is, we haven't got anyone . . .' She goes into a prolonged moan about the lack of management time put into co-ordinating the work of the chiropodists. They never know, when they are turning up to see a patient, if a colleague has beaten them to it. And another thing . . .

Jackie tries hard to look sympathetic but already she's thinking about dinner at her sister's this evening. Is it still on? She should ring her. She feels guilty when the woman trudges off to the lifts, but then she mutters to herself. 'Like the bloody number 9 bus, never one when you want one, and then . . .'

The pharmacist, a slim man with a roguish face and a nudging smirk of a smile, is leaning on her desk, watching the chiropodist go. He has a sheaf of forms he is pretending to fill in.

'Have you seen Mr Clark?' Jackie asks.

'Yes, nice man, not as barking as I thought he would be,' says the pharmacist. 'And how are things today?'

'About normal,' says Jackie.

'Bit of a change all this, eh, Jackie? Must be nice to have electric lights, not having to keep the donkey on the treadmill all the time?' He grins broadly. The pharmacist is always trying to tease her about her last hospital, one of the smaller south London units swept away in the last round of closures. Jackie gives him a withering look.

Yet all the time Jackie has had one ear on the door behind her. In there the patient who has been weak with heart disease for months is just fading away, propped in a chair by the bed, wrapped in blankets. Every so often, as the door opens and the nurses go in, discreetly checking the man's condition, the other patients get a glimpse inside: the wrapped body, the ash-grey face, the laboured, inconstant breathing, the wife sitting beside him, waiting. Jackie knows he is slipping away, she has seen it too often before. Experience tells her he will go this morning. She discusses the practicalities quietly with her senior staff nurse: when he goes, the body will have to be certified. That means making sure there is a house officer available to do the paperwork, remember not to upset the other patients.

For the rest of the morning Jackie just sits, contemplating, doing her paperwork, waiting for the time, discreetly moving on the boisterous and the good-hearted. She doesn't have to wait long. When the wife finally emerges in tears, Jackie is up to meet her immediately. The pharmacist, who was discreetly testing a student he had in tow, moves quietly down the corridor.

The nurses keep watch. Even if they heard the cries, the other patients do not emerge to investigate. Most are eating lunch. Jackie leads the wife down to the relatives' room while a health assistant makes her a mug of tea. A staff nurse pins a 'Do Not Disturb' notice on the isolation room door.

Ten minutes later Jackie returns, and calls a house officer to certify death. The body must be prepared, a son has turned up – just minutes too late – and there is paperwork to be done. Jackie is torn between sadness and relief. But she knows that whatever she feels, she must just work through it; she still has half her shift to go. She sits at her desk, thinking of all the coronaries and heart disease and strokes and suffering she has seen. The quick and the slow. She has suffered with all those she saw suffering. Their cries have knocked her very heart. But all she can do is her bit to help, whatever else is going on around her. Whatever the politicians do, whatever the managers and doctors do, you just get on with it. With a smile.

Down the corridor, another patient emerges from the lavatory, whistling incongruously.

32

Just before her treatment ends, Carole witnesses a row in the Oncology waiting room. June is sitting there in her fur coat, telling the other patients about her private health plan, insisting that her lump would never have been found on the NHS. After she is called in for her treatment, another patient complains to the woman at reception that June has been seen first because she is going privately. It's not true, says the woman, you all have allocated times, there is no difference between private and NHS down here. 'But those of us on the NHS just have to wait longer!' retorts the patient. Others from the waiting room back him up. Oh, God, it's come to this, thinks Carole.

When she finishes her treatment she goes back to see the consultant. He asks: does she mind? There is a *Panorama* crew outside who are making a programme on cancer services and they would like to film their conversation. Yes, she would mind, actually. She feels guilty but enough is enough, she doesn't want any cameras. Fuck the cameras. You cannot move in hospitals for cameras these days. Don't they know people are dying? Of course they do. The hospital might as well just video everyone and sell it, or set up their own channel for pervs and voyeurs.

The doctor gives her another examination and says, you look fine. Come back to the clinic every six months for a check-up. You shouldn't get pregnant, because if the cancer does return, you might have to undergo chemotherapy. If nothing returns in the next five years . . .

She vows she will go every three months. She lives with the fear every day.

33

There is a small fire in the basement. Little damage is caused, but no one is sure how it started. Security is stepped up.

34

John leans back further and studies his visitor watchfully through pale grey eyes. 'If given the option,' he gulps, 'I would swallow ... lots of pills ... and end it ... of course I would ...'

When one gets to the end of one's life, he continues, one gets more philosophical. He fought in the war. He has seen things. He is old. He can accept his fate. If he was a young man, he would be angry. 'It begins ... to dawn ... on me ... as each day passes ... the value of my life ... to me myself ... is becoming less ... and less,' he says. 'It is my life ... why can't I ... decide what I want ... to do with it ... it is my life ... the one thing that ... is mine ... and mine alone.'

He is not a religious person, he adds. He does not believe in an afterlife. 'What is faith?' he asks his visitor. 'Define it ... it is the acceptance ... of theory ... without any support ... of factual evidence ... I don't know ... And furthermore ... I would suggest ... mankind ... will never know.'

A faint smile plays on his lips. He is enjoying the conversation, the chance to talk about things which no one else will broach with him. His eyes move quickly, his face, ever immobile, with its furrowed parchment skin, takes on a lizard-like intensity. He is riding the conversation now, reining it round, in control, no longer the passive martyr of a hundred different arrows of debilitation. What does anyone know about death? *This is what we fear ... nothing to think with, nothing to love or link with.* Surely no more than he who sits contemplating it every day, anticipating its firm embrace.

He tells his visitor a story he heard when he was small. Once there was a two-dimensional world much the same as ours.

One day a man in the market-place saw a spot appear on the ground. He watched it grow bigger and bigger, and as he did so a crowd joined him. Soon the spot filled the whole of the market-place. Then slowly the spot began to diminish, bit by bit, until eventually there was nothing left. Everyone said: what was that? They couldn't comprehend, in their two-dimensional world, that it was a sphere passing through.

Now maybe in our three-dimensional world, John continues, there is evidence of a fourth. We call it time. We see evidence of its effects, people age, speed can be judged, but we do not understand what it is.

His visitor looks confused.

'So I am content . . . to believe that . . .' The engineer pauses, and his visitor wonders if he has lost the thread. Then, as the ventilator fills his lungs, he starts again: '. . . there must be . . . some sense to it all.'

So John sits and waits. While he talks, a plump West Indian cleaner in a blue housecoat climbs the ramp and asks the visitor, can I share the bench? OK, says the visitor, we're just chatting. The cleaner has a wide white smile which she broadens as she settles down. She gives John a long look.

'Oh, yes,' she laughs. 'He's my boyfriend, arntcha? Hee hee hee . . .' And she gives a girlish giggle that wraps around the two men like a much-loved fleece.

THE BEST OF ALL POSSIBLE HUMAN ACHIEVEMENTS

The first essential is to have your nerves well in hand.

Sir William Osler, medical scholar (1849–1919)

We expect the world of doctors.

John Updike, introduction to *The House of God*, by Samuel Shem MD

1

One night a woman walks into A&E wearing nothing but a fur coat. She is in agony. When the sister asks what is the matter, she opens the fur coat. She has a frozen trout thrust up her, stuck hard, which she cannot remove. The fish's gills, as sharp as the barbs on any arrow, lock it firmly in place. Soon the same story is being spread in every hospital, a key part of that sacred little corner of popular hospital mythology: what did you find stuck up the patient? Hoover nozzles, lightbulbs, fruit and veg, telephones, a bust of Napoleon. Don't ask. Usually it is men, but women can join in too. The public never loses its capacity to surprise.

No one can quite recall what happened to the patient, or how the fish was finally removed. When the sister who treated her went to work overseas, her friends brought some pertinent mementoes to her leaving party. Sales of trout shot up that day.

2

Early morning on an old ward, the sun just pushing through the long windows.

'I want two coffees.'

The harsh voice cuts the calm. Patients look round. Pushing

the tea trolley over to the bed, Constance gives the woman a long, appraising stare. She is used to rude people. The woman, a visitor, middle-aged and foreign in appearance, possibly Italian, is sitting beside an older woman's bed. Her mother. She doesn't even look up. Look at me then, thinks Constance.

The rest of the ward carries on with its lying about. Patients eye each other casually, looking to find who's sicker, slowly getting used to sleeping with strangers. Kathy, Constance's friend, is clearing up further along the ward. She watches the confrontation, a smile playing over her thin lips. I'm not going to say anything, thinks Constance. Just give the woman her coffee and walk on. She moves slowly but with purpose, handing out the cup without saying anything, pushing the trolley on to the next bed. She has her thin shell of indifference to protect her, but her brown eyes are smouldering.

The next morning the same woman is back early. It's not yet seven. She must be staying in Gassiot House. When Constance arrives, she is already checking on her mother. Constance watches the two women warily. Only when the younger woman leaves does Constance fill her tea trolley and start the rounds. By the time the woman returns with a young man, her son, Constance has finished and is searching for her broom. She hears the woman ask a nurse: 'Can I have a cup of coffee for my son, please?' It is a sharp, shrill voice, edged with the confident expectation of having wishes fulfilled and orders followed.

'There's the domestic,' says the nurse, gesturing down the ward to where Constance is unpacking her equipment. 'Ask her.'

But already Constance is through the door at the end and into the staff lavatory. She sits down and thinks, no way, I ain't doing it, not for the earth. It's that woman's attitude. By the time she goes back, the woman has got the nurse to do it.

Constance is a cleaner. At 42, she is rounder than she was, not too tall, with a pretty, cherubic face and a halo of tight black curls. She works in the second NHS. If the first is full of bosses and surgeons and chairpeople who think of progress gained and objectives achieved, the second is inhabited by everyone else: the workers who just get on with it, who face daily rudeness and sparse resources and eternal crisis. At times, the two can seem worlds apart.

Getting angry is not in Constance's nature. She never rushes anything, it's not her style; she is cautious in her movements. With good reason, too, on account of her hernia operations. No more lifting and stretching. That's what stopped her being a home help, that and the walking. So much walking. She used to start in Catford and end up in Bromley, then one of the people she was home-helping for would want their shopping done in Catford so she would have to go back. Then others wouldn't want their supper till six so she'd have to go out again. Oh, don't get her started.

No, it wasn't for her. The money was good, though. She brought home £150 a week, then if she did another four hours on Saturday and another four hours on Sunday it was £50 on top. No kidding. But the walking. She hates walking. She'd rather take a couple of buses in to the hospital every morning from her home in Catford, because she can't bear the thought of doing the five-minute walk from Waterloo station.

She came over to Britain from Jamaica with her mum when she was six. London is her real home now. She has tried going back to the Caribbean for long holidays but she misses the bustle and excitement of London. She has got a man with a good job, she has got three nearly grown-up kids, she has got somewhere nice to live, what more do you need? Well, money would be nice. She does the Lottery off and on, and once won £10. One day her numbers might come up. One day they did, but it was the Wednesday draw and she doesn't play Wednesdays. That would slaughter some people but Constance, she's happy. Hospital work isn't bad, mostly she likes it, she gets £4.64 an hour for a 39-hour week. It's more than she got when she worked for a cleaning agency. That's how she got the job. Did it first for an agency, then got offered a permanent position. She worked at Guy's for a bit; it was the same kind of people but the work was a bit harder. Here, she is left to get on with it. It's good.

Most days she gets up at five, has half a cup of tea and heads for the bus stop with her kids still in bed. She gets one bus in Whitefoot Lane, then another in Peckham. That usually gets her to the hospital by twenty to seven. She puts on her cleaner's coat in the changing room downstairs and clocks on at seven. The night nurses don't hand over till 7.15, so they are just beginning to get their stuff together. Constance puts on her rubber gloves and empties all the bins of medical waste: bloodbags, dressings, wrappers. The breakfast trolleys come up at 7.30 and then Constance does her first tea round of the day. She deals with everyone and everything. Puts hot chocolate in the microwave for the fussy ones, doles out tea and coffee to others, listens to people's worries. Just occasionally she's even been known to get cigarettes from the student bar for some lucky patients.

Most of them stay in bed. In the old days they would have had to get up, but a lot of patients now are too sick to move. There's not much to get excited about. The food? Well, you can order a sandwich if you want, but most people need hot meals. One morning the breakfasts came up with just one sausage and one piece of bacon per plate. What happened to the egg? asked Constance. Oh, the chef overslept this morning so you can't have any eggs, she was told. She thought: one man oversleeps and the whole hospital has to do without eggs? It's crazy! Lucky it was only breakfast, really. Times have changed. She remembers when she was in hospital having her kids she would get boiled egg and toast every morning, real nice. Now, if the patients have cornflakes, they don't even get enough milk to go on it, and tiny little things of butter and marmalade. That's terrible. She thinks they probably enjoy the tea more than the breakfast.

Once the first tea round is done she gets her broom and does the floor. Then she wipes the table, cleans up round the beds, does some more sweeping, and wheels round the tea trolley again. Five times a day it goes round. If she forgets the biscuits at three she has to go back to the kitchen to get them. At 10.30, Kathy, the other cleaner, comes on and Constance gets half an hour break. Most days she takes a cup of tea down to the staff room. The cleaners asked for a kettle for the room but no one would buy it for them. If it's on the ward, you get one. If you're a cleaner, tough. You can buy it yourself. No one wants to do that: you never know how long you are going to be in a job, and what with the hospital having three blocks, not everyone uses the staff room anyway. Just another little indication of where you come in the pecking order. Last, really.

That said, she doesn't blame the supervisors for being tough. She has no problems with them, but a lot of cleaners always seem to be off sick. Just in February, she did 36 hours of overtime as cover. She doesn't think they are bunking off. It's just the pressure. On some wards there is only one cleaner; they may be ill, but they still come in to work because they know they are needed. Then they get sicker, and when they go off, they go off for a long time.

She has got a supervisor called Greta and a manager, Greta's boss, called Chris. She hasn't really worked out why she needs two but she guesses that if she doesn't get satisfaction from the one she can go to the other. That's about as much management as she sees. She doesn't even know what the chief executive looks like, let alone his name. He might as well be on another planet.

Another supervisor started last week. He came up to the ward about six times on his first day, on his own personal efficiency drive. Constance was working down one end of the ward and he popped up at the other, waving away, like a gleeful bystander at a royal procession. So she waved back, figured it must keep him happy.

'Just checking you've got everything you need?' he said, smiling.

He must be keen, thought Constance. If he is going to do this every day, my arm is going to get tired.

3

Picture the scene: Tim Matthews sits in a private meeting on the Guy's site, smiling blandly, giving nothing away, smoothly thinking figures. Opposite, the project manager for one of the contractors involved in the new Guy's hospital building is explaining for the fourth time why it isn't his company's fault that the costs have run over and everything is late. Matthews listens. The man opposite, maybe he is broad and weather-hardened, with a face walnut-wrinkled with worry, just talks, as if talking could build a ladder out of the hole he is in. Matthews spends a lot of his time contemplating that hole, hearing this talk again and again as he tries to work his way round a building commission that appears to have gone disastrously wrong. By this stage, the arguments are spinning around everyone's heads like the hook of a bad pop tune.

Too much of the Trust's management time is being spent trying to unravel an unworkable past and tie up an uncertain future. It has inherited a building project at Guy's, commissioned by the old regime, which has swiftly become an embarrassment. It has also been ordered to get private capital involved in any further major projects it is planning. So Matthews' days are mapped out, rushing from meetings with contractors trying to sort out the massive cost and time overruns on the Guy's building, to meetings with construction companies trying to interest them in funding a new women and children's hospital at St Thomas'. The irony is not lost on him. As both projects progress, he swiftly decides that neither the old nor the new ways are good enough.

He asked to see the service plan for the new Guy's building on his first day as head of the joint Trust. To his surprise, he found there was neither any plan nor any revenue assumptions for how, once it was completed, the new building would pay for itself. There was also no clear documentation of what the contract position was with the building, how much it had cost so far, how that compared to original estimates, and how much the projected overrun was likely to be. The only list suggesting what specialisms might go into it had been drawn up five years previously, before the review of London health services. The project, which had been started at the end of the eighties and only finished four years late, in 1997, appeared to many to be an organisational shambles, and worse than that, a pretentious folly, with far too many waiting rooms, vast atria and real palm trees shipped up from wherever you ship palm trees from. Cornwall? The Scilly Isles? Bermuda? He didn't want to know. Fifty years of National Health Service expertise and it had come to this. That was what happens, whispered the managers, when you let doctors design a hospital on their own. Another firm of management consultants had to be brought in just to tot up what the overruns would be. Matthews had already negotiated with the Department of Health, when the Trust was set up, that the Government would pick up the £160m tab for the project – that was only fair, as its commissioning was the fault of the old regime – but the building seemed to overwhelm anyone associated with it. Just as a mysterious copper-eating disease put paid to its new pipework before it had even opened, so many of the building's contractors simply fell apart. Profits warnings were issued. Subsidiaries were demerged. Likewise the whole process of negotiation and renegotiation over cost ate into the Trust's senior management time. NHS time. NHS money.

The Private Finance Initiative was just as debilitating. Matthews had got the doctors behind the idea of a new women and children's hospital on the St Thomas' site. But the Government insisted that, before any application was made to the Department of Health for cash to fund the building, the project had to be put out to tender in the private sector. The idea was to demonstrate whether public or private funding represented the best value and best transfer of risk. It was similar to the principle of leasing new trains for the Underground off a third party. Construction companies would be told what the hospital wanted. They would then pay for the building, and recoup the cost by leasing the facilities back to the hospital and using the site for other purposes – hotels, car parks, whatever. It seemed a sound idea, it had already been discussed as a way of funding a new teaching building for the medical school on the Guy's site. But it was complicated. Sometimes a hospital's priorities just weren't compatible with those of big business.

Matthews and his team spent two years working on the process. Field work had to be completed on what others had done. Documentation drawn up to show to interested parties. Presentations made about what the Trust wanted on the St Thomas' site and what the opportunities were. A firm of management consultants were appointed to help with the process. An ad was put in the *European Journal* announcing the scheme. Three consortia, two UK-based and one American, expressed interest. More paperwork had to be completed. And all the time the chief executive and his team were asking themselves: with the political instability surrounding health in London, who is really going to commit themselves to something of this magnitude? The Americans backed out. The Trust invited detailed responses from the two consortia left, both headed by construction companies. The consortia sent in more piles of paper, and came in to give their own presentations. They said: this is our concept of how the site would work. Matthews' team looked at the numbers. They didn't add up. How is this going to work financially? You say these are your financial requirements, but we know from operating buildings like this that it doesn't look right. Others from the hospital who saw the designs thought they were unworkable: operating theatres in the wrong place, criteria and priorities all jumbled up.

Another consortium dropped out. The last one hung on. The

Trust spent more months working the proposals through. It compared them with its own proposals for a publicly funded scheme. It drew up a document, analysing what value for money or transfer of risk was gained, and submitted that to the Department of Health and the Treasury. It was decided, eventually, that not enough was gained. The private consortium was furious, but decided not to make an issue of the affair as it hoped to win other PFI deals elsewhere in the country. Around £750,000 and an incalculable number of management hours later, the Trust was back where it had started.

Like the new Guy's building, it became another rod for the management's back. Wasting time, flushing away money, fiddling around with the electrics in the corner while the patient was arresting on the table.

4

Describe the pain. You can't exactly. It's like a violent, vicious form of indigestion, but higher. It's like a steel string twisted tight across your chest, but worse. It's like a cold, giddy sickness breaking over pain-stabbed limbs. You feel nauseous. You lose your sense of direction. You think you are going to fall. You don't know what it is.

Mary has just gone out to pick up some tablets in Newton Abbot. George has parked the car, bought a ticket for half an hour – he is going to collect some shoes from the cobbler. They are pensioners, they have to be careful with their money. Even a short shopping trip could end up costing more than they can afford. See you back here in half an hour, he says.

He knows something is wrong when she doesn't come back.

He has that feeling. It has been nagging at him for weeks. 'Oh, she's a tough old bird,' he tells friends, but he knows she hasn't been looking herself, he can see the worry lines etched round her eyes. Sometimes you feel right as rain and then it all starts falling apart. That's what growing old is. Fit as a fiddle, then . . . Last year she had a stroke, completely out of the blue, no warning; she was helping her daughter clear up some water from the washing machine when she nearly keeled over. Afterwards she couldn't remember anything, her short-term memory was completely wiped out. She spent a few days in hospital and slowly it all seemed to come back together. Things aren't exactly the same, but at 76, you are grateful to get back to something close. You can walk, you can talk, you can look after yourself. Tough old bird. George is only 66. 'I'm her toy-boy!' he likes to joke. But then the pains in her chest started. The doctors gave her a nitrate spray to ease them, yet George is worried. He had a bypass operation ten years back. He knows the signs. Not Mary, he hopes, not my Mary.

That moment in the car park seems to last forever. Maybe there's a queue at the chemist's, he thinks, but he knows it wouldn't normally take her this long. Perhaps she's chatting with a friend. Yet she wouldn't leave him just waiting, not if she said she would be back in half an hour. She isn't like that. Just as he has made up his mind to head for the chemist, he sees her, standing dazed at the other side of the car park. She looks awful: pale, disoriented, frightened, unsure of her feet, turned in on herself, as if she is fighting some exhausting battle deep down inside, and losing. He runs over and grabs her with both hands.

'What's the matter? Mary, what's the matter?'

She can barely speak. She whispers something. He cannot catch it. He helps her over to the car and tells her to wait. Think. He has got to do something. Think. The GP's surgery. It's just around the corner. Can he leave her? She might not make it if he tries to take her all the way.

'Stay here,' he says slowly and clearly, looking deep into her frightened eyes. 'I am going to get help.' He sees the gratitude flash out above the struggle. They have been married 40 years. He tells himself: she's a tough old bird, it's OK, she's a tough old bird. He runs round to the doctor's surgery. Thank God, he is there.

'You've got to help me, please, it's my wife, I think she is having a heart attack.'

The doctor comes out and together they help Mary back to the surgery. He tells her to stay still and phones for an ambulance to take her to Torbay Hospital. They put her in a ward. They keep giving her tests. George goes home that evening not knowing what is happening.

It doesn't become much clearer over the next few days. No one is sure what to do. Was it a heart attack? Should she have an angiogram? The consultants discuss it. George visits every day. They tell him that maybe a bit of clot from her stroke has got to her heart. At least, he thinks that's what they mean. It seems to him that there is a lot of uncertainty, not just his own. Then they say to him: she should have more tests, she can't have them here, we think she should be transferred to either Bristol or London, which would you prefer? He talks to Mary about it – both agree London. They remember something in the local papers about a heart surgeon in Bristol being dismissed for low recovery rates. It has nothing to do with the tests, but mud sticks. They wait.

Eight days after she is admitted to hospital, Mary is told there is space at St Thomas', 200 miles away. She will be taken up by ambulance tomorrow.

5

Take me to the place where you go, where nobody knows . . .

Fried bread.
  Bacon.
  Eggs.
  Sausages.
  Kippers.
  The cardiac anaesthetist sniffs at the breakfast on offer in Aida's Café. His face, dark and round and airline-pilot good-looking, is puckered into a little frown over the bacon on the hot plate. He pauses, uncurling his tall body. He looks slim, but is beginning to carry just a little bit extra on his belly. Perhaps he is thinking of his weight. Perhaps he is thinking of the heart surgery on his list today. Before he can even choose the kippers, Aida, standing the other side of the counter, has put one on a plate for him with a grilled tomato. She gives him a big grin that lights up her whole wide face as she hands the plate over. Favoured customer. Always has the same.

  The café is no more than a hole in the wall, a small, windowless room wedged between the operating theatres in the North and East Wings, up on the second floor. There is enough space for two tables, an assortment of plastic chairs and stools, a long bar of hot food, tea, coffee and juice, and Aida. The room is so tiny that the dirty dishes and cups have to be stacked on a trolley outside. Inside the air is thick with food-steam and the fug of murmured conversation. It could be a cabbies' canteen, or a tiny transport café. But many of the men eating here are among the hospital's biggest earners. They sit in their blue theatre pyjamas, with their head caps pushed back and their masks dangling, drinking tea with their registrars and shovelling down a quick breakfast. This is their sanctum, their refuge when their lists go 'pear-shaped', or they get a quarter of an hour off while a junior sews up, or are thrown the chance of some two-minute tea while another patient is brought down. They talk of hospital gossip and job appointments, schools and politics, anything they want. There are no patients or managers to eavesdrop. This is their space.

Outside in the corridor an official sign in the standard typeface, white lettering on brown, discreetly says 'Aida's Café', named after the broad-grinned Philippine who runs it. Chris Aps thought that was a nice touch. As the clinical director in charge of the operating theatres he gets to sort out the signs, as well as organise who is working where and what equipment goes into what space. He also has to find out why whatever it is that isn't working, isn't working. It's the bit of his job that he really doesn't enjoy, the bit that has completely changed his relationship with the other doctors he works with. Suddenly, to them, he's not a doctor any more – he's the management. Then someone says something, or makes a snide remark, or bangs on about some piece of equipment he has tried for months to replace, and he feels really pissed off. He gives up a lot of free time to be clinical director – time he could just as happily devote to his private patients, or to writing learned papers, or simply to having an easier time. Instead, here he is, 51 years old, head of department, respected cardiac anaesthetist, and he's got senior house officers hassling him to sign their car parking forms, and all he wants to say is, Oi! It used to be *you* did things for *me*! Not any more.

One thing he is sure of: by the time this generation of junior doctors get to his level, they won't put up with the amount of work he has to get through. Twenty hours of operating a week, on-call duties, management, teaching and out-patient responsibilities. Sometimes he can be up all night operating on a emergency and then have to go straight into his regular list the next morning, sleepless. Of course, he still fits his private patients in. Like so many other consultants he works ten sessions out of a nominal eleven at the hospital, which gives him roughly half a day free for private work. In practice it means he operates for the NHS two days a week, splits the rest of the time between managing the department and seeing patients, and squeezes the private work around that. By the end of the week he is always knackered, drifting off to sleep at home in the middle of *News At Ten*.

But there are up-sides. Organising the theatres for the hospital's new cardiothoracic centre was one of them. Designed to take over the heart and lung work of St Thomas', Guy's and the Brook Hospital, now closed down, the centre is a huge improvement on past facilities. The chief executive was keen to throw money at it (cardiac surgery is a good cash generator) and all the research showed that the bigger the unit, the lower the mortality figures, so bigger really was better in terms of care. Bigger units simply attract better expertise. Nothing like feeling the hot breath of peer-group competition to keep the scalpel hand steady. So Aps drew up plans for refurbishing the theatres and sorting out the wards, and developed an ingenious answer to the log-jam that always blocks cardiac surgery: the problem of beds in Intensive Care. If there are not enough beds to take the patients after their operations, surgery has to stop. If surgery stops, money stops. If money stops, managers want heads to roll. So he asked the obvious question: why put cardiac patients in Intensive Care? Instead he developed a new idea: a nine-bedded overnight intensive recovery unit which would operate within the main post-operative recovery unit. The logic was simple. Intensive Care is hugely expensive to run. It uses lots of expensive equipment, employs lots of expensive nurses and administers lots of expensive drugs. But often the patients don't need that level of care. An overnight recovery unit – offering a scaled-down version of Intensive Care facilities – works fine for most of the cardiac patients, especially if you can get them off the ventilator as soon as possible.

To outsiders it seems rather obvious: a halfway house between a normal ward and Intensive Care. But it is more complicated than that. It requires 'fast-tracking' the patient so that 'extubation' (getting the patient off the ventilator) can be achieved as soon as possible. That involves using shorter-acting drugs, keeping the patient warmer during surgery, using vasodilators (drugs which dilate the blood vessels) to speed up the warming process, and a host of other things. Aps is proud of what they have achieved: a gleaming new unit, a higher through-put of patients, some good publicity about ground-breaking work at St Thomas'. He even got Damon Hill, the racing driver, to open the unit – very appropriate, he thought – and showed a junior health minister round. The minister was impressed. Cardiac surgery is one of the fastest-growing areas of medicine. Yet as fast as hospitals unblock the patients' veins, they are always finding their own systems gummed up with emergencies in Intensive Care. This showed a way of bypassing the problem. It had a neat symmetry.

But this morning even Aps' system has gummed up. He was in at seven, after a quick stop at the London Bridge Hospital to check on the private patients he operated on yesterday, only to find that this morning's list was on hold while they tried to clear the beds in Recovery. There was a Caesarean that had gone wrong from Obstetrics, there were emergencies from A&E in Intensive Care. By seven-thirty, still nothing had shifted. At eight he decided it was no good hanging around in theatre, he would get something to eat.

The worst is the waiting. Cardiac surgery always starts early, simply because it used to be a long-winded procedure, eating up whole days. Now it is routine, each bypass operation often taking no longer than three hours. But they still start early, because tradition dictates it. So the theatre nurses have already been in for half an hour and right now they are sitting around being paid to do nothing simply because Fate has intervened and blocked the beds. Nothing you can do about Fate, he reasons, as he pokes his kipper. Beds need staff, and you can't keep an endless supply of staffed-up, free beds on the off-chance there might be an emergency. It is one of the points that the businessmen and politicians and economists never seem to understand about hospitals. It is a juggling act. Things go right and things go wrong. You have to balance what you need now against what you might need later. And occasionally Fate nudges your elbow.

A nurse pops her head round the door of the café. 'You're on. We've got two free beds.'

6

The Admiral, chairman of the Trust since 1995, the man brought in to steady the ship after the chief executive's sexual peccadillo became tabloid news, sits in his first-floor office opposite Parliament, conducting a meeting. His wavy grey hair is blown back like a fluttering spinnaker, his little dark eyes are screwed tight in concentration, and his demeanour is as clipped and assured as if he was still in uniform. Many of the hospital staff make no secret that they find his appointment bizarre: 40 years in the navy, straight out of running the Trident missile programme into chairing Britain's biggest hospital trust. He also heads up the UK Atomic Energy Authority and has in the past run the Portsmouth docks. It is the stuff of sitcoms, they say, shaking their heads – all unfair, of course, but hospitals are hotbeds of malicious gossip.

If the Admiral has heard any of it, he doesn't show it. He exudes confidence in his own command, and runs his meetings with reasonable firmness, somewhat in contrast to the chief executive's occasionally rather glib lassitude. There are times, too, when the Admiral's decisive manner is a positive advantage, not least in dealing with criticism of the Trust, which the chief executive just seems to smile through. If this contrast in styles annoys either of them, they don't show it. They persevere. No one outside the two of them knows how well they really get on together.

The Admiral doesn't speak to many journalists. He has a well-worn mistrust of the media, understandably so, given his involvement with Trident and nuclear power, but just occasionally, like now, he consents, reluctantly, to give an interview. He describes the situation at the Trust, what he feels it does successfully, where it falls down. He says that morale at the Trust is a problem, but he puts that down to the anxieties of merger and the complexities of unpicking the past. In particular, he says, the long-running difficulties over the new building project at Guy's, now finally completed, have sapped staff's confidence in the management team. But it's not fair, he says.

'Trying to sort out the debris of the past to find a way forward is not easy. By and large the past determines where you are, and most of it determines where you are going. If you have a contract it is going to run forward. If you have a lousy contract it is still going to run forward. Trying to sort it out is incredibly difficult, if not impossible. You can only band-aid it, you are never going to give it a new heart. It is very easy to criticise other people in hindsight, more difficult to put yourself in their position ten, seven, five years ago. Anyone can look at it with hindsight and say, if only they had done this. That's what the media do. They say: oh, you shouldn't have driven down that road, then you wouldn't have had that accident.' And he shrugs dismissively.

7

Matt Tee gets a call from Carlton, the local ITV station. It wants to send a news crew round to shoot an item on the new Guy's building.

The reporter is a woman, young, maybe 27, blonde and dippy, wearing a sharp black suit that sets off her pristine bob. Butter wouldn't melt in her mouth. Tee takes them on a tour of the new building, the largest new hospital development in south London for 20 years, and shows them its offices and treatment rooms, its atria and palm trees, its airy walkways and fancy brickwork. The reporter says: 'Can I just have a talking head to say how nice it is going to be in the new building?' And she bats her eyelashes as if to say: I would be ever so grateful and it's not much of a request, really, is it?

'Yup,' says Tee, 'how about me?'

'Oh, that would be fine,' she says. 'Just stuff like where the benefits to patients are going to come from and that sort of thing.'

'Fine,' says Tee.

So they shoot it on the lawn outside the PR office at Guy's. She asks him, all cutesy, how nice is it going to be. Very nice, he says, running through the facilities.

Then she says: 'What about the cost overrun?'

Then she says: 'And what about the carpet millionaire not wanting his name on it?'

Then she says: 'And aren't you being investigated by the National Audit Office over the way the building project was managed?'

And all the time the cameraman and sound man are grinning

away like malicious monkeys in a safari park intent on whipping off his wipers.

Tee takes it all in his stride. He has prepared the answers. He knows the game. He pours oil over his answers, whipping them creamy-smooth and insubstantial, but patiently correct. That's what he likes about his job, he can busk it when he sniffs trouble, he doesn't have to go running to the chief executive saying: what do *you* think? That's why he thinks the chief executive, who rarely appears before the cameras, is a great manager. He delegates superbly.

8

George gets a shock when he sees Mary again. She is lying in a pool of blood on a bed in a cardiac ward. She had a bad night. Earlier in the week the doctors inserted a catheter and sent coloured dye winking round her veins under local anaesthetic; she felt nothing as the dye tunnelled away while the doctors X-rayed its progress. Three badly blocked arteries round her heart, they said. Yesterday she had angioplasty. A little balloon was inserted on the end of a catheter and then expanded to remove the blockage. It didn't work. Mary wasn't sure what happened next but the doctors seemed to struggle for hours. When they finished, and removed the catheter from her groin, the bleeding just went on and on. She lay all night with a compression weight on the wound to slow the flow. When she was moved the next morning the blood had soaked through her nightie and her sheets to the mattress below. The consultant came in to apologise for the trauma. Sometimes, he said, cupping his chin with his hand, these things happened. He seemed genuinely upset about the discomfort she had suffered, as if it had piqued his professional pride.

George hears all this second-hand. He has just come up on a day visit, driven by his son-in-law. He wanted to get a lift in the ambulance that took Mary up, but then at the last minute he was told there was no room, they had to take another patient. He thought about going up by train and staying at the hospital, but they said she might be back in a couple of days, and anyway, they don't have much to live on, just a pension, they have to be careful what they spend. It's a four-and-a-half-hour drive up to London from Newton Abbot. He is getting on. He isn't sure he could manage it on his own.

He asks the ward sister when Mary will be sent back to Torbay. Probably tomorrow, she says, we'll just make sure she is OK to travel, ring and check tomorrow. George goes back south that evening thinking everything must be all right. He rings up the next morning. There's been a change of plan, he is told. We are keeping her in. She is going to have bypass surgery as soon as possible.

9

If you want to annoy an anaesthetist there is a simple way. Just ask him: *do you have to be a doctor to become a wotchamacallit?* Imagine how he feels. Eleven years of training and they ask me that! And it happens all the time.

Putting a body to sleep, and holding it there, floating and insensible, is a dextrous skill. Upon it much of modern medicine relies. To many it is also a mysterious craft, a voodoo mix of chemicals and gases, clotters and thinners, vein-openers and closers, warmer-uppers and cooler-downers. An anaesthetist has to practise that craft in the knowledge that the slightest slip, the merest miscalculation, can maim or kill. An anaesthetist, as everyone in a hospital knows, has the capacity to leave dead bodies all over the place. The fact that anaesthetists' accidents don't happen all the time is rarely remarked upon, nor are anaesthetists routinely congratulated for it. It goes with the turf. Hence their manner. They are generally warm and meticulous men (nearly always men), with a highly polished bedside charm, well versed in the art of reassuring the patient, who lies quaking in fear, dreading the operation. Sometimes they are not always honest men, for in their off-duty moments they will also tell you: don't have surgery unless you absolutely have to, it's not worth the risk. Then they will smile and change the subject. The patient just concentrates on the smile.

Chris Aps loves his profession. He sees himself as each patient's personal physician; more than that, he describes himself as each patient's personal pilot, there to fly them through the operation and make sure they land safely. Nor is it just an idle metaphor: he has been a pilot for years. He flies from Biggin Hill, just in borrowed planes, for – as he likes to point out – you never quite earn enough as an anaesthetist to buy your own. He picked up the bug from an ex-RAF friend of his dentist father who took him flying in a Gypsy Moth when he was just 16. Thirty-five years later, for his 50th birthday present, Aps' family bought him another trip in a Gypsy Moth to commemorate it. But what he really wants to fly is a Tornado. Running an operation, he thinks, is a bit like flying a Tornado. Pilot up front, navigator behind. He isn't sure if the surgeon would like being just a navigator. He would probably have to give that simile a bit more thought. Others in the hospital find his boyish enthusiasms intriguing. Apart from being an excellent doctor, he has been married a few times – the sort of behaviour which always raises eyebrows among colleagues in any institution.

He rings for the first patient to be brought down. She is old, 76, with unstable angina. He looks at the notes. They have done all the usual blood tests and X-rays. They have tried angioplasty, sticking £2,000-worth of tiny balloon into each vein and gently expanding it, hoping to ungum the works. No success. Not enough oxygenated blood was getting through. Even if it had worked, she would probably have been back within a year. Now instead she is going to have the full operation. Triple heart bypass. Two veins stripped from the leg and a mammary artery rerouted from just behind the breastbone. It is standard stuff. There are six to do today. He looks at the list and who else is operating. Two in theatre one, two in theatre two, two in theatre three – if the beds become available. So somewhere in the hospital six people are lying, waiting, starved, believing today is their day. Better not let them down. He just wishes people understood more about heart surgery. There should be a book on it in W.H. Smith, he thinks, explaining everything in plain man's English, answering all the questions. It really isn't anything remarkable any more. Most of us will probably have it at some stage in our lives.

The patient is wheeled in by a porter, with a ward sister behind him. They are standing in the little anaesthetics room off theatre three, filled with drugs and cupboards and a long, wheeled table on which the patient will be operated on. It is barely big enough to hold the patient's bed and give enough space for the anaesthetist to squeeze round. Aps says hello to the patient. Mary smiles up bleakly, her grey hair scraped back, her eyes slightly disoriented and frightened. She appears resigned, her loose, pale throat offered up to the harsh light as she lies back. She has slept well – every patient gets a small sedative the night before the operation to stop them worrying – but already seems exhausted by the anticipation.

'This is Norman, my assistant,' says Aps, introducing the short, fleshy man who is standing behind him. Norman raises a pudgy finger and a big, friendly smile, the sort you use to pacify the terrified. In his other hand is a clipboard. 'Can I just check your name?' he asks. 'Do you have any false teeth? Have you had anything to eat and drink in the last 12 hours? Do you . . .'

Aps takes her hand. 'Mary. Can I call you Mary? How are you? All right? Any pain? No, good. What have we got here?' He runs his free hand under her body, feeling the extra mattress on the trolley-bed. He looks at the sister enquiringly. 'An extra mattress for special people?' The sister nods, and murmurs, not sure if the question is addressed to her, 'Yes, for frail people.'

'Just lie still and we will slide you across,' says Aps.

They slip a slide under her and pull her gently on to the table. Aps takes a syringe from the counter behind him. 'I'll just give you something to sedate you, Mary,' he says, injecting her slowly. Mary's eyelids flutter slightly. Norman starts attaching little pads to her side, wired up to the monitor at the end of the table.

'I'm just going to give you a little bit of oxygen, Mary, it's good for your heart.' He holds a mask over her face, she breathes deeply. 'You will wake up wearing one of these, so don't be worried.'

Norman is still working quietly beside her. A cannula, a thin, sharp white tube, has been inserted into her arm and a drip bag of saline solution attached. Another line is attached to her wrist through which Aps can monitor her blood pressure. The midazolam, a Valium-like sedative, is beginning to work. Mary's head lolls. Aps starts inserting cannulae into her neck through which he can administer drugs and monitor pressure in the central venous part of the heart. Routine cardiac surgery will involve as many as 30 drugs or more. Around a third are just to put the patient out then bring them back. Others affect the heart, the brain, the kidneys, the circulation. Then there are the various antibiotics, and the analgesic to mask the pain, and the steroids to mask the effect of the cardiac pulmonary bypass machine that will pump the blood while the surgeon slices and sews the heart. Many of these drugs can be administered or altered at any stage during the operation. All work in tandem with the gases and vapours that the patient might also be inhaling. That is how the anaesthetist flies the patient. And different anaesthetists use a different mix – that's their style.

247

Norman connects the cannula in the wrist to a transducer which flashes the pressure readings to a small screen at the end of the table. Aps inserts another into the jugular vein with deft, practised precision, like a small boy assembling a favourite Airfix kit. He has four cannulae in the neck now – some anaesthetists operate with as many as six. Mary is snoring, oblivious to the intrusion. The final touch: Aps slips an incontinence pad under her head to catch any blood. It is always better, he says to himself, if the patient wakes up feeling clean and nice, and not looking as if she has been butchered.

Then he administers the final doses before the operation starts: a powerful painkiller and drugs to induce unconsciousness and paralysis. As Mary's breathing falls he pulls a mask over her face and starts to hand pump the lungs, slowly, regularly, using a small rubber balloon, all the time gripping her throat with his right hand, keeping it upright. They wait for full paralysis to set in. If he stopped pumping now, Mary would die. Then swiftly, dextrously, he removes the mask and forces open her mouth with a steel laryngoscope, through which he inserts two tubes down her throat, a fat one to the lungs, a thin one into the stomach. Smoothly the ventilator takes over her breathing.

Just then a nurse pushes open the swing door from the corridor. 'We've received a major incident alert,' she says. 'There's been a train accident at Victoria.'

Aps groans. It is too late to stop the operation, but the alert means that all the other operations will have to wait. The hospital must keep its theatres clear for emergencies. He looks at Norman. 'I think the technical term here is S.H.I.T., don't you?' He ties the tubes in place with a bandage knotted over Mary's mouth. Norman wraps Mary's arms in soft woollen gauze to keep her warm. Aps slips an elastic-edged plastic hat round her head. They stop for the briefest moment to check their work, like a couple of couturiers inspecting a difficult new design, then wheel her into the theatre, where the surgical registrars are waiting.

'There you are,' says Aps as he attaches her to a ventilator. 'Still alive.'

The registrars, all earnest eyes and belligerent brows, smile behind their masks.

10

George gets a lift up to London again that morning. He wants to get there by lunchtime – they have told him Mary's operation will probably take place in the afternoon. One o'clock will give him plenty of time. He has mixed feelings about the hospital. He likes the fact that it is in London, he knows it is a national centre for cardiac surgery, he feels Mary is in good hands. But it is so far away. No one can visit her. And it is so large and impersonal and, well, maybe a bit rough. There has already been an incident with a health assistant when Mary was being taken for her angiogram. She told him about it last week. It was a Tuesday. She was nervous. She wasn't allowed to eat. They starved her one day, then put back the test another 24 hours, so she was starved for a second. When she was finally told it was time, she was so grateful she started burbling on, just for reassurance and a bit of friendliness, to the assistant who was wheeling her to the lift.

Finally she asked: 'Am I your last one tonight then?'

The assistant scowled at her and then looked straight ahead. 'I don't give a shit,' she muttered as she kept pushing. Mary was shocked, and didn't say another word. George was furious when he heard and reported it to the sister, who said she would sort it out.

These things happen, George reasons; he would still rather be here than Bristol. But he'd liked the Brompton where he had had his operation ten years before. Things seemed a bit friendlier. There was not such a mass of different people every-where.

11

'What's that Oasis song you are always playing?'

The senior surgical registrar looks up quizzically from where he is working on Mary's chest.

'"Don't Look Back In Anger",' says Aps, his voice slightly muffled by his paper mask. The registrar bends down again, focusing through the long black magnifying lenses attached to his spectacles. They look like Barbie-doll binoculars crudely glued to his glasses.

'That was it,' he says.

'Haven't got it here,' says the anaesthetist. He is fiddling with a large ghetto-blaster in the corner of the operating theatre. He slips on a CD. *Yellow Brick Road* by Elton John.

When are you gonna come down . . .When are you gonna land . . .

'I liked the Oasis song. Just doesn't feel the same without it.'

Aps shrugs.

The registrar is studying the rectangle of chest visible through the surgical drape. Mary has been stripped, cathetered, painted with an iodine-based antiseptic from neck to toe, and redressed with a large green sheet. The exposed flesh is covered with a fine, clear plastic film which will protect the wound from any bugs that might sweat out of her own pores. Her head lies to one side, mouth stuffed full of tubes, face covered by another sheet propped up on rods. Her legs poke out of the bottom. A senior house officer works on the left leg, slicing from knee to ankle, searching for veins to strip out for the heart. The other registrar, leaning over her chest from the right, prepares to split her breastbone. Aps, who likes to stand, watches carefully. He has set up his bank of machinery behind the patient's head. He takes up his position, legs slightly apart, equipment on either side, screens to the left of him, dials to the right, fibrillators, defibrillators, pacers, cardiovascular drips. He looks as if he is about to pound out a fugue for some long-since-defunct pomp-rock band.

'OK if I start?' says the registrar. Aps nods. The patient is awash with drugs now. A little trolley of ampoules and syringes waits down by the anaesthetist's right hand. A tussle of tubes emerge from the cannulae inserted into the patient's neck. A plastic bag under the operating table slowly expands with urine from the catheter. The anaesthetist is ready for take-off.

Slowly the ventilator pumps her lungs. Aps watches the readings carefully. The music has become a low drone as he thinks. Sometimes, when they are really tired or hauled in to do an emergency in the middle of the night, the heart team dip all the theatre lights except for the main spots over the table, and really pump up the volume. Anyone stumbling in would go, whoa! Where am I? Some weird nightclub?

They were in at 2 a.m. last Sunday, all hauled out of bed for an emergency that came in from Kent. They operated until seven in the morning. It couldn't wait. If they had delayed, the patient would have died. They needed the music to keep them going. *Hello, hello, it's good to be back, good to be back.* Other times, when it is really serious, the music goes off, and their voices drop to low and clipped. That's when you know you are up against it.

'Hello, Chris, how are you?'

The surgeon walks in, a compact man, in his mid-40s, serious-looking. He carries a sheaf of papers and a *Times*. He nods at the rest of the team and wanders round the back to scrub up. The operation will be done in three parts: opening up Mary's chest and leg and extracting the veins to be used for the bypass; sewing the veins in place on the heart; and closing the chest and leg. The surgeon's expertise is only needed for part two. His assistants do the rest.

The registrar is already into the chest, prising apart the ribs with a giant steel retractor. The bones, hinged on the spine, part reluctantly, like an old clam. The surgeon watches approvingly while he ties on his green apron and chats to Aps about lists and equipment. Do you want to know the effect the internal market is having on my patients, he asks. The anaesthetist feels a rant coming on. Everyone likes to rant at him; after all, he's a clinical director. I'll tell you, says the surgeon, my whole operating list is now being drawn up by a computer program which works out who comes from which health authority, what form of contract that authority has with the hospital, and who must be done first to prevent penalty fines kicking in. Whatever happened to medical criteria?

'It's like having 60 different purchasing bodies, all with different contracts which give them different priorities,' he goes on. 'I am effectively running 60 waiting lists with the GP fundholders on top! It should be a one-month wait for urgent patients and three months for routine. Now we're lucky if we do the urgent in three months and the routine in 12. It's bloody ridiculous.'

Aps looks sympathetic. No one knows what to do about the ever-escalating demand for heart surgery. In the old days GPs just told patients to live with angina. Now they put them on the list for surgery at whatever age, in their 50s, in their 70s, even in their 90s. The Government set a target of 350 bypass operations per million head of population, and already in their patch of south London it is running close to 300 and rising. The new unit will do 1,500 this year. At around £5,000 a go, that is a lot of money swishing through the system.

Slowly the team numbers grow. A quietly anxious perfusionist – the man who will run the heart-lung machine while the surgeon operates – takes up position on a stool behind his equipment.

The machine will suck in Mary's blood, turning venous blood into arterial blood, before pumping it round her body again. He checks everything is in order: the cooler heater to control the blood temperature, the gas blender to supervise the gas mix, the small plastic sack which collects the blood sucked out of the wound during the operation so that not a drop is wasted. While the anaesthetist flies the body, the perfusionist will keep the propeller turning.

The surgeon plans to strangle the heart into a tiny tremble before beginning work on it. Each vein takes around six minutes to sew in. In between each bout of sewing they will start the heart again, shocking it with the little black paddles of the internal defibrillator. Meanwhile the perfusionist will drop the body temperature, putting it into hibernation, so it needs less oxygen. Already the team has started plumbing in the lines that will bypass the heart and leave the surgeon free to work. Mary is now just a blood-soaked hole of gristle and muscle and fat and bone. In the centre quivers her heart, that fearful engine of tissue that looks too tiny to power so large a corpse. They finger around it gently.

The surgeon moves to the patient's right, replacing the registrar, who shifts to the other side of the body to assist him. He stretches out the veins stripped from the leg over his fingers. The veins look thin and white-rubbery, streaked in blood and limply lifeless. Unusually, one of the veins has a small clot in it. The surgeon frowns as he flushes it with heparin saline solution to clear it. Sometimes everything seems to fall so neatly into place – God surely anticipated cardiac surgery, doctors joke, that's why he put so many non-essential veins in the body – and other times the unexpected catches you out. Who would expect a stripped-out vein to have a clot in it? He works quickly to clear it, and then starts sewing it in with little flicks of a tiny curved needle. Aps watches carefully. He has seen it so often he could probably do it himself, but he needs to keep watching so he can see if the surgeon hits a hitch.

'Excuse me.' A nurse pops her head round the operating theatre door. 'There's a message for you from the Harley Street Clinic. They want to know if they can take out all the drains in your patient.'

The surgeon sighs as the team exchange a glance.

'It's not even my patient,' says the surgeon, half apologetically. He briefs the nurse, never once looking up from the vein he is working on. 'By the way,' she says, 'the Victoria alert is cancelled. No one was badly hurt.' The team shrug and the door flaps shut as she goes back to the phone.

'Rewarm, please,' says the surgeon. The perfusionist nods. He has to be warned in advance that the vein is nearly in place.

'Clamps off,' says the surgeon. The blood begins to flow through the patient.

'Yup, thanks,' says the perfusionist.

The surgeon pulls out a swab from under the heart and squeezes it. The squish of blood dribbles back into the cavity.

'Back to you,' says the surgeon.

'OK,' says the perfusionist. The heart shrinks to half its size as the blood flow bypasses it. It quivers gently. The surgeon, leaning over close, cuts another tiny hole with his scalpel.

I will crush your heart to ease your pain.

Someone turns up the music. Its mundanity slices through the taut concentration in the theatre. *B-B-B-Bennie and the Jets . . .*

Aps watches the numbers on the screens as the surgeon defibs the heart. The figures flick up and down. Up to 110. Down to 78. He can coax the rate either way with drugs which work on the nerves controlling the heart. One nerve that makes it beat faster. Another nerve that makes it beat slower. Accelerator and brake. He is flying smoothly while the surgical team patches it all up on the wing.

The surgeon finishes the last bit of sewing. Aps winches up one side of the operating table to get the body at the right angle for the surgeon. Barely a word passes between them. They wait to see if the new plumbing works. They have done it so many times before. Aps keeps the little table of drugs close to his hand. If there is a hitch, this is when he will earn his money. You never know how the heart will react to being starved of oxygen during the operation. He has seen the fittest hearts go down. At the other end of the patient the senior house officer works remorselessly on the leg, sewing up the knee-to-ankle slash with the rapid professionalism of an expert upholsterer. What looked like butchery is now being pulled together tightly with swift jerks of the needle into a close-lipped long red scar.

The heart works. The bleeding stops. The surgeon barely acknowledges it, simply turning away to let his registrar close the huge wound. Using a thick steel hook he punctures the chest bones and pulls them back together with eight twists of wire. A short tube sucking blood out of the wound vibrates noisily as it hits air.

'Can you reduce the suction, please, it's making a dreadful noise.'

A nurse nods. Behind the patient's head, Aps prowls by his machines. Some of the equipment looks old and well used. Much of it desperately needs replacing, something he has fought for, but he keeps being told there just isn't money available. Other anaesthetists complain regularly to him. He has told them: if they feel it is unsafe to go on with the operation, then they must not proceed. He even tried to squeeze a million pounds out of the Special Trustees. As a rule they won't fund replacement kit but will bankroll innovation, so he used a bit of lateral thinking and said he needed new gas delivery systems, rather than replacement anaesthetics machines, and put in a bid. He thought he might get something but he was smoked out by the panel of crusty old codgers who pass judgement on every bid. A surgeon said he didn't need the kit. Didn't need the kit? He should come and operate here instead of bumbling around on committees. The anaesthetist knows he didn't really handle it well. He will have to get better at the politics. What he should have done, he thinks, was put in a bid for 44 machines for anaesthetising kids with heart disease and cancer. Kids with cancer always works.

By now the registrar is bandaging up the wound and they are tidying up the patient, removing the sheets, cleaning away the blood. The music goes off with a click, breaking the spell. As the trolley-bed from next door is wheeled in, the outside world rushes back to envelop them. The patient is transferred gently on to the bed and connected to a new, smaller monitor which records her ECG reading, blood pressure and oxygen level.

'Is she OK?'

'Yeah. Blood pressure 153 over 38.'

Aps ventilates Mary by hand again, squeezing 100 per cent oxygen into her lungs via a small rubber bag. He grabs his notes and follows the trolley as a theatre porter wheels it down the corridor towards the recovery room. He trundles the bed into a vacant slot next to a new bank of machinery waiting to be plugged in. Aps chats to the sister in charge, squidging round the bed in his white boots. Mary slowly begins to come round, her heavy-lidded eyes fighting the weight of the anaesthetics, her body's nervous system just beginning to get the first intimations of trauma through its call-and-response system. The sister bends down and talks softly in her ear. 'You've had your operation and you are in recovery now. We are going to give you something to help you sleep soon.'

Mary has landed.

Aps smiles as he walks slowly back to Aida's Café. One down, another to go. Maybe just time for a cup of tea before the next one. Too late. A nurse stops him to tell him more beds are freeing up and they have brought the next patient down already. No tea then, but he seems to tread a bit more lightly. It looks as if all the patients scheduled for bypass surgery will get their operations this morning.

He gives the next patient a cheery hello as he enters the anaesthetics room. The patient, a pukka-looking pensioner with a military moustache and sad-looking eyes, nods back. Norman has already taken his details.

'OK,' says Aps, slipping into his patter, his manner as cool as if he is just casting off the painter for a little dinghy-sail, 'I am going to give you an injection now, a bit stingy like the dentist but not as nasty as that.' He slips a cannula into a furrow of saggy old flesh round the patient's wrist and smiles reassuringly.

'Comfortable? There. That's good.'

'Let's get it over with,' says the patient. 'I can't wait.'

12

It's not till George checks with the ward sister that he finds out the operation has already taken place. Mary has been moved to a recovery ward. She looks drawn and wan, her face sideways down on the pillow, unconscious, her skin a yellow shade of white. She still hasn't come round properly. George sits with her and holds her hand. 'Trust you to beat me to it,' he says, chuckling softly in her ear. He remembers that when he had his operation, she sat with him for days, talking to him, holding his hand. He remembers her saying: the last faculty you lose and the first you regain after anaesthetic is your hearing. Now he wants to do the same for her. He wants Mary to hear his voice when she comes round.

He is still there at 11 p.m., whispering and squeezing. One of the nurses encourages him: go on, she says, she will hear you, keep trying. So he does.

'Come on, love, open your eyes, let me know you are all right,' he whispers. Just then her lids flutter and her eyes open three times, then she sinks back to sleep. George smiles. Bed, he thinks. He has booked a room in Gassiot House, £2) a night, reserved for patients' relatives and family. It's nothing special, just a bedroom with access to a shared bathroom and kitchen, but it is all he needs. He tells the nurse he is going, and she slips him a piece of paper with the ward phone number on it. If you are worried and can't sleep, she says, you can give us a ring. We'll tell you how she is doing. Thanks, he says, I will.

When he gets back to his bedroom, he is tired but his adrenaline is pumping so hard he cannot keep his eyes closed. By 3 a.m. he is looking for the internal phone in the corridor. He dials the number on the piece of paper he was given.

'How is she?' he asks, muffling his voice, hoping not to disturb any light sleepers.

'She's perfectly all right, no problems at all,' says the nurse. 'You get to bed again.'

13

A fire breaks out in a lift shaft at two in the morning on a Saturday. The operating theatres which run between North Wing and Lambeth Wing have to be closed after thick, sticky smoke coats the walls. A&E is shut to major trauma cases for four hours till an emergency operating table is established in East Wing. The whisper goes round that an arsonist has been at work. What sort of person would set fire to somewhere so close to a building stuffed with bed-bound patients? A sick person. Two years earlier someone sabotaged the electricity supply at Guy's. No electricity, no ventilators. Luckily the back-up generators kicked in before the Intensive Care unit was affected. No one speaks about these things much to outsiders. If the press wanted to whip this all up . . .

Everyone just does their job, same old thing. The site practitioner gets on the phone to patients who are due in on Sunday.

Nearly 400 operations are cancelled over the next fortnight. Out-patient appointments have to be moved, doors replaced, ceiling tiles renewed, walls cleaned, smoke-damaged machinery overhauled. That is the strength of a good hospital. People just get on with it.

14

Most of the time Constance is pushing her broom, she is thinking, what am I going to cook for the kids tonight?

The patients are the good bit. There is one at the moment, an old lady, probably around 80, who always says 'Coffee, two sugars, please,' whenever Constance appears. She's a character. Coffee and two sugars. Oh dear, it always cracks her up. Then there is Andrew, the ward comedian, you don't want to believe anything *he* says.

The ward is a mixed one, 27 beds, ladies up the top end with their own shower and toilet, men down the other. Those who are well enough get up and chat, but most stay put. After a bit, everybody knows each other – well, you would, wouldn't you? They all wake up together, don't they? It's a bit like *The Waltons*. Are you up, then? No one seems to mind that it's mixed. For some it has advantages. The other day a patient and her boyfriend were caught in the loo by a nurse up the ladies' end. They had both gone in together and forgotten to lock the door. The nurse opens it and what does she see? Well, you can guess. He had his trousers down, she was up on the basin, pumping and a-grindin'. Very athletic. The patient, she's 24, sickle-cell, has to have a pregnancy test every week now. No one else saw what they were doing but the whole ward got to hear about it.

Now when Constance is doing the toilets she knocks real loudly first. She is always a bit disappointed when they are empty.

Some patients you get attached to, and it hurts when you lose them. With a few, you just know they are going. There was an old man who Constance liked, who she chatted to one Wednesday night, he looked all right, he had only come in with bed sores. The plastic surgeon had been round and said: 'I'll do him Friday.' But come Thursday morning he was going, you could tell. He looked right through Constance. She thought, that's not right. Next minute everyone was rushing around. She thought, oh Lord, oh Lord. He died later that day. His wife was there, crying. Constance had tears in her eyes too. At one point she thought the whole ward was crying, he was such a sweet man.

After her mid-morning break Constance gets out her mop for the first time. She has half the ward to do, Kathy does the other half. Half the ward, two side rooms, two toilets, bathroom, shower. She starts at eleven o'clock and has got 45 minutes to do it before lunch comes up. She is mopping away and a visitor comes up. 'That's how I bust my hip,' says the woman sourly, pointing at the wet floor. That's how I bust my hip, I ask you. The woman looks like she's been sucking lemons. Constance sighs and goes to fetch her WET FLOOR sign. Then a doctor walks straight through where she has just cleaned. Isn't he looking? Some doctors are OK, but others . . . she cannot understand them. They walk around like God and don't even notice your existence. The nurses are great, though. They are all pretty quiet, until they have their parties. They had one before Christmas, doctors and nurses, and when Constance came in the next morning, she found part of the ceiling had caved in. No one owned up to it. Probably students, everyone said. Sure.

Next, she does the loos while everyone is eating – it is the only time they are empty. She has to scrub hard to get rid of the dirty feet marks. She can't understand where the dirt comes from. After all, the patients never go out. Who's bringing it in? As soon as they put their feet down the marks are there. And if the loos are dirty she has to clean them again and again. At times like that she thinks, I can't do this job long-term, I've got to find something else.

15

Everyone has their gripes. Working in a big hospital is a high-pressure business, but it is also, first and foremost, a people business. You need people skills. And sometimes, it seems, the higher up the job ladder you go, the less likely you are to see those skills.

'The surgeon I am working for is really difficult,' says the house officer on one surgical team. 'You get no support for anything you do, you get shouted at when anything goes wrong, the pressure is continual. It is so undermining of your own self-confidence. I mean, I am 30, I have worked before, and last week I was in tears every morning before I went in. When I'm at work, I can hardly control myself. I know I am doing the job badly because I am so affected by what is going on.

'The thing I most resent is that it is interfering with my private life. I've lost confidence, and I don't believe that I should be so undermined. And if it makes me, a confident 30-year-old, feel that, what does it make a lot of the others who go through the job feel?

'I think being a woman does come into it. There are three of us house officers on the team. Two of us are women. The other woman who works with me doesn't drink, and she gets completely ignored by the rest of the team. Basically, you can't not drink and not go out on a surgical team. She just doesn't exist as far as they are concerned.

'The guy, on the other hand, is very St Thomas'-minded, he's joined all the right clubs and goes to all the right dinners, and the senior members of the team are more comfortable dealing with him. We tend to divide up the patients, and even when it's one of ours that the team is looking at, they ask him.

'But it's the little things that get you. I'll give you an example. Last week I was told to get the X-rays for the patients to be operated on the next morning. One set was missing, the X-ray department was closed and didn't open till 9 a.m., the operating list started at 8.30 a.m. so I said to the senior registrar, could we swap the first two patients round so we've time to get the X-rays in the morning? He said no, it was absolutely out of the question. But all the patients had been starved the night before, it wouldn't have affected anyone except the porter who went to get them.

'So of course at 8.30 a.m. I got bleeped and asked why the X-rays weren't there. I told him again. He said go to X-ray and find them. I went to X-ray. There were about five people there, who'd just got in: two consultants, two secretaries and a cleaner. I explained what was happening and they were all really helpful, they all looked for the scan, even the cleaner! I just thought, why are these consultants having to do this, just because they feel sorry for me?'

'Meanwhile the other woman house officer was summoned to theatre by the surgeon, who said he wanted someone to shout at. He started screaming at her, shouting, why aren't the scans there? They should have been done yesterday! You're useless! You get nought out of ten for your job! I mean, that's just abusing your staff.

'And the ward rounds, they are just ridiculous. Sometimes we have nearly 17 people trailing round, seniors, juniors, physiotherapists, nurses from the ward, maybe some other consultants. I mean, it is a huge body of people that walks up to each bed. If I was a patient I would be absolutely terrified. And what tends to happen is that the more doctors you have there, the less responsibility anybody takes for talking to the patient. And it is very rare that on this ward round any patient gets talked to. You laugh but I am not exaggerating. It is intensely embarrassing.'

'You know, some of the surgeons are great, but . . . well, most people won't speak about it because often you are only there for a few months before you go on to something else. You just keep your head down. I am not bothered, because I don't want to make my career here.'

16

George stays at St Thomas' for a week. His days swiftly fall into a routine. Visiting Mary in the ward, popping into Shepherd's Hall restaurant for a cooked meal, spending the afternoon with Mary again, chatting, sometimes taking some photos. Her ward overlooks the back of Waterloo and the Eurostar terminus. They spend the days watching the trains come and go, dreaming of trips they can make, places they still have to see. Then George makes some sandwiches for tea. Mary gets better every day, but he begins to worry about the cost. Even at £20 a night, the bill for his room in Gassiot House quickly mounts up. £120 is a week's pension.

Eventually the doctors say she can go. George is relieved. He takes her down in a wheelchair to where their son-in-law is waiting with his car. The nurses have taken the dressings off her chest. The scar has already begun to heal nicely. On her leg, though, there are still patches where the wound is weeping. It is a long drive home – four and a half hours, too long, thinks George, for someone who has just had open-heart surgery. Mary looks exhausted at the end of it. At times like that he thinks, maybe it is just too far to go for an operation. Too out of reach of friends and family. Maybe she should have had it in Bristol. Better still if she could have had it in Plymouth.

She has to keep taking her painkillers. It hurts like hell if she coughs or sneezes. It feels like her whole chest is splitting open again. She has to grab a cushion to herself and hug it tightly if she feels a sneeze coming. It's agony. George remembers when he was given painkillers after his operation. I don't need these, he told the nurse then, I am not in any pain. You soon will be if you don't swallow them, laughed the nurse. George smiles at the memory. Mary is also sullen and weepy after the operation, just like he was. George remembers that he cried buckets. He was told it was because his heart had been touched. Actually touched. Some people gave him funny looks when he explained, but he knew what it meant.

The wound on Mary's leg takes longer to heal than they thought, nearly a month. She still doesn't look right to George. Her pulse is racing, sometimes hitting 140. He gets the GP to check her into Torbay Hospital for more tests, and the doctors start talking about giving her an electric shock to bring her pulse down again. They explain that you can get an irregular heartbeat after a bypass operation. It is usually corrected with medication, but sometimes that doesn't work. So then you have to try shocking it, stopping the heart for half a second at the exact moment it fibrillates, in the hope that it gets going again in the proper rhythm. Mary doesn't really want to do it but she has to do something. Sometimes her heartbeat goes so fast it actually seems to move, making her jump on her seat. The doctors press her for a decision.

But nice things happen too. One day there is a knock at the door and a man they have never met before is standing there, asking, can he have a word with Mary? It turns out he is a friend of a neighbour and had a heart bypass operation some months back. He wanted to come round and reassure her that it was going to be all right. While they have tea and a chat, George gets his photos out from the packet on the sideboard where he keeps them. Photos of the view from Cheselden Ward out over the Thames towards the Houses of Parliament. The seat of power. A beautiful view. You can't beat it, he tells their visitor.

17

After two fires in a month, Matthews uses the Trust newspaper to appeal for vigilance. Staff must report to Security anyone acting suspiciously. Everyone must be careful not to leave waste in unauthorised areas. The police continue their investigations, but there is little expectation that anyone will be caught. The firestarter knows his or her way round the hospital, and security in the buildings is becoming increasingly difficult to enforce. For years, the hospital has been targeted by professional (and unprofessional) thieves. Nothing is safe. Toasters, televisions, fridges, all disappear regularly. Bags get pickpocketed. Drug cabinets get jemmied apart. Security staff have their hands full just dealing with the fights. It is the same in hospitals all over London. The bigger the institutions become, the more they seem to teeter towards anarchy. Things fall apart, the centre cannot hold. Politicians mouth fine words but appear powerless to help.

18

For the 1997 general election Tee writes a detailed protocol listing what is and isn't acceptable political behaviour for Trust staff on hospital premises. No party badges on uniform, no party posters on Trust property. Tee himself spends his spare time campaigning for Labour, even gives up a weekend to support his friend Stephen Twigg, who is fighting Michael Portillo. People wonder whether Tee misses being more closely involved with Labour's ascent to power. He says he would have been uncomfortable with the cynical pragmatism of New Labour, but few doubt that he understands the public-relations possibilities.

Before the 1997 general election is even announced, Tee is doing the rounds of the political parties, spelling out what Guy's and St Thomas' have to offer for leader visits. He even shows representatives of the Labour and Conservative parties round. It pays off. One Tuesday, halfway through the campaign, he gets a call from Tony Blair's office. The Labour leader wants to take over a visit to St Thomas' cancer services planned for Chris Smith. On Thursday. They have less than 48 hours to organise it.

The head of cancer services, a plump, shrewd man with a reassuring smile, gets the same call. Within a couple of hours he has no fewer than four Labour Party organisers and a Special Branch representative sitting in his riverside office, discussing what's on offer. He is easy-going about the intrusion. A long-time friend of Smith's – he was treasurer of the Student Union at Cambridge while Smith was president – he has been advising the Labour Party on a new strategy for breast cancer treatment for the past year. He has no illusions about the politicians' interest:

breast cancer is a big lobby. In terms of new cases of cancer, it is less common than lung cancer, but because people who have had it tend to live for longer, the numbers mount up. At any one time there are a quarter of a million people alive in this country who have had breast cancer (as opposed to about 40,000 with lung cancer). Add family and friends, and that is a lot of voters with personal experience of the condition. Margaret Thatcher announced the national breast cancer screening initiative for the 1987 election. Tony Blair announces a £10m injection into breast cancer services for the 1997 election. Politicians on the same wavelength, looking for votes.

The meeting passes amicably enough. Blair's team agree he should visit the ward and the radiotherapy department, Outpatients and the chemotherapy area. They discuss the order they should do it in, they look at it from the security point of view, they work out the best places for photo-opportunities, they decide who is going to hold the lift. Then they decide that there will be a question-and-answer sesssion for staff, either on the lawn or, if it's raining, in Central Hall by Queen Victoria. The photo expert hums and haws over that one, not sure about the stained-glass backdrop (wrong image). If they do the question-and-answer there, maybe they will have to switch the positioning round.

The next day, while the head of cancer services is walking the wards, talking to staff and sorting out which patients would be suitable to meet Blair, the haggling begins. One of the Labour Party organisers rings up the public-relations department and says they need children for the photos. 'Aren't there any cancer kids? We have got to have cancer kids.' Not on the St Thomas' site. The organiser goes back to her boss. They will do it without cancer kids. Nothing is left to chance.

On the day, the visit starts smoothly. The red Rover carrying Tony and Cherie Blair glides round the hospital's riverside walk, right up to the front entrance. The chief executive, the medical director and the head of cancer services are waiting to meet them. Matthews shakes Blair's hand. He notices that Blair's eyes are glazed, his gestures smoothly affable, a professional campaigner. They visit the wards and the treatment areas, accompanied by a posse of sharply dressed Labour Party underlings and a television crew which will supply film for the news pool. The patients love it – anything to relieve the mundanity of hospital life. The Blairs light up with big smiles and meaningful handshakes. Everything runs to plan until the question-and-answer session. Pharmacists, midwives, senior nurses and consultants turn up. No one is wearing a white coat! They all look like managers! 'We've got to have some nurses and white coats!' hisses one of Blair's team. Tee's public-relations staff scour the North Wing for junior doctors and nurses.

Tee's prime concern is to make sure no rabid Trots jump out from behind pillars at the wrong moment. When he is asked by a journalist what the hospital gets out of it all, he replies, without hesitation: 'It says that, when the man who is about to be Prime Minister wants to visit a hospital in London, he chooses to go to St Thomas'.' It's a good day for PR. Public relations, that is.

After the Blair visit is shown at length on *News At Ten*, Tee's counterpart at King's College Hospital rings him up.

'You jammy bastard!' he says. 'How did you manage that?'

'Yeah,' replies Tee. 'I think Blair just wanted to come to a real hospital, don't you?'

It's just a joke, but he savours the moment.

19

Constance has little time for politics. She buys a cheese sandwich and a Lilt from the newsagent and sits in the staff room, eating slowly. Other workers come in and out. They chat about the overtime pay. It's not time and a half, but time and a quarter. Stingy? Tell them about it.

It's a good mix, black and white, West Indian, Portuguese, Cockney. Everyone gets on. The only trouble they get is from visitors. One cleaner tells Constance how she was using the phone the other day and a visitor called her a fucking bitch. What for? The cleaner shrugs. Maybe because she doesn't speak very good English. Maybe because she was using a phone. Maybe because the visitor was a bigot. It is the second time it has happened to her, she says.

After lunch Constance has to finish what she started earlier, polishing the floor, then clearing out the nurses' changing room, cleaning their toilet, then the passage where the lifts are. Invariably there's a patient standing there in his pyjamas, puffing quietly on a cigarette, looking at the notice which says, please do not smoke here, go to the visitors' room. Constance sweeps up the fag ends.

She does the tea trolley one last time and checks her bins again. She clocks off at five to four, catches the 53 to New Cross, the 136 to Catford and the 134 to take her home. She likes the buses, and whatever anyone says, there's no real difference between them and taking the train. One girl at work leaves at the same time as her and is only just coming out of Lewisham station as she goes past. She thinks about what she is going to make the kids for supper as she waits for the buses. Sausage and chips from the freezer? She cannot remember what's left. Maybe she'll make chicken curry instead, only she forgot to defrost the chicken this morning so she'll have to stop and buy some more.

At 5.30 she's home. She likes to get the kids' supper ready by 6.30 at the latest. She eats with them, and more often than not is in bed by eight. One night she went to bed so early she woke up at 11 p.m. and thought it was morning.

20

Shortly after Tony Blair is elected Prime Minister, Tim Matthews makes a presentation to senior staff, analysing the new government's health strategy. He sums up: public health will take a more central role with the health authorities, the internal market will be reined back, there will be greater focus on collaboration rather than competition, and greater openness and public accountability.

'The changes in service organisation and delivery on which the Trust is already embarked provide us with a unique set of opportunities to both shape and lead this new agenda,' he says. His tone is uncharacteristically upbeat. In fact, no one knows what changes the Government are going to make, or how they are going to enforce them, or how it will affect individual trusts. But right now, every hospital chief executive needs to be seen waving the flag cheerfully. Especially if they want government money for new projects.

21

The full Trust board – thirteen in all – sit round a long table, studying a thick wedge of papers. This afternoon Matthews, looking relaxed in a well-pressed red-striped shirt, is to present formally his plans for the Trust's next big building project: the women and children's hospital on the St Thomas' site. His team have prepared a business case, local politicians have been softened up, the media sounded out. The £114m project, which also involves the development of new cancer and renal centres, and the transfer of Guy's A&E service over to St Thomas', is Matthews' chance to make a big mark on the Trust, not just sorting out someone else's new building, or unruffling feathers for an unwanted merger. This is something striking, something permanent, something the chief executive can stake his career on. The PFI option has gone. Now it's government money or nothing. If the Department of Health and the Treasury refuse to back it, he will probably leave. He will have done five years in the job by 1998. Maybe it will be time to move on.

The Admiral sits in the middle of the table, running the meeting. Already there is a whisper among senior staff that the new Labour government will be unlikely to renew his contract – a new chairman, more congenial to the new, non-competitive approach to the health market, is on the cards. If he has heard the rumours, he doesn't show it. His demeanour is as assured as ever. 'Chief executive's report. Tim?' he says briskly.

'Right, um, well ... First I guess you will have heard we had another minor infection outbreak at Guy's. It makes it all the more important that we recruit an infection specialist at consultant level. We have tried advertising but we only got one applicant last time. I think it was because of the way the job was structured. It is clearly important that we fill this post as soon as possible ...'

The other directors nod in agreement. As well as the chairman and seven executives, there are five non-executive directors present, appointed to represent the public's interest and drawn from the private sector. Given the range of their backgrounds – solicitor, accountant, public relations executive, businessman (all appointed as part of the previous government's efforts to wrench hospital-running away from local politicians) – you might suppose that some of the proceedings might be tough for a few of them to follow. The meetings can last for hours. Discussion can be arcane. Even the one health professional amongst them, the principal of UMDS, who used to help manage Guy's, appears to have difficulty maintaining concentration. By the time Matthews is halfway through his report he is already looking up at a far corner of the room, clearly deep in his own thoughts.

The topics float by, like leaves on a pond: appointments, franchises, protocol and procedures. The sub-committee reports, the reconfiguration reports, the performance reports. 'We have had a very good month for revenue,' says the finance director, a tall man with a stern moustache and the smile of a hungry wolf. 'We have also had lower costs than anticipated. We are still receiving money from GP fundholders from last year who queried their bills. In terms of expenditure, the clinical group have overspent rather modestly by their standards. We have also had a rate rebate following a long appeal over our rating assessment with the district valuer, and we have still got another judgement to come. By contrast I have to report that the full-year forecast position is not as healthy as the year to date . . .'

The number of operations being bought is down, income from commercial services is likely to decline, there are whispers that the transitional funding promised by the Department of Health to help with the cost of reorganising the Trust is going to be removed and paid to other London hospitals who have deeper financial crises.

'I have argued that they have no case for doing this,' says the finance director, 'and certainly not halfway through the financial year. They accept that but say there are greater forces at play.'

The Admiral scowls. 'This is ridiculous. They cannot act retrospectively, letting us spend money and then telling us we haven't got it. They cannot penalise us for being efficient.' He shakes his head. Matthews pours himself a glass of mineral water from the bottle on the table. No one says anything. Their thoughts are plain. Even if you get your finances sorted out, you can be kicked in the teeth with these kind of on-the-hoof decisions. Waiting lists are getting longer, health authorities have less money to spend, the hospitals are performing fewer operations than they want to, winter is coming up. It doesn't bear thinking about. Eventually the Admiral moves on to the next item of business.

'Tim, do you want to introduce the new plans?'

'Thank you, Chairman. I thought I would take this opportunity to present to the board the Trust's Full Business Case, as it is known, our plans for development of the St Thomas' site following the opening of Thomas Guy House at Guy's.' He gestures to the thick file in front of each director. 'Let me start by running through the reasons for what we want to do.'

He talks through the main criteria, educational, strategic and service. Clinical: the current configuration is not providing the optimal clinical service that the Trust is capable of. Educational: many of the clinical departments do not have the size and weight to be first-class university hospital departments unless merged. Financial: the Trust started life with £18m of transitional funding in order that it should find savings through merger, a strategy born out of the findings of the Tomlinson review. He reminds them of recent history: Tomlinson in 1992, the Trust's formation in 1993, the publication of Lambeth Southwark Lewisham Health Authority's acute services strategy just months later, the start of the PFI process within the Trust in 1995, the funding of the new cardiac centre in 1996, the collapse of PFI by 1997. None of it is news to the board, but it sets everything in context.

'So, with the commissioning of both Thomas Guy House, and the cardiac centre at St Thomas', the Trust has already made significant progress, but further major restructuring is required if the Trust is to meet its service, financial and academic objectives. This Business Case seeks the capital funding required to deliver the Trust's strategy. The capital sum, £114m, is large and requires careful justification. This is set out in this document.' He taps the file in front of him.

'OK, there are four very talismanic things we can deliver: first, a single centre for acute and emergency care. Second, a new centre for elective care. Third, London's first integrated women and children's hospital. Fourth, major unified specialist centres.'

He presses his fingers together, forming a pointed arch with his hands. 'So that,' he says, summing up, 'is what I want to deliver out of this. Clearly the case has to be strong and robust, but it is important that we as a board are clear that what we want out of this is not just strong financial arguments but something we can hang our hat on that will really provide something worthwhile . . .'

22

August 1997. Diana, Princess of Wales dies in a car crash in Paris. The nation mourns. What can be built in her memory? What sort of project would provide a fitting memorial to her special talents and interests? Matthews and his team, like hospital executives all over Britain, have an idea.

23

Joe can't believe it. They have been told to come in at 8 p.m. and there's no one about.

'Hello! Hello! Is anyone there?'

Anna sits in a chair by the sixth-floor reception, suitcase at her feet, her hands resting on top of her beachball stomach. She is wearing glasses and a long raincoat. A small frown wrinkles her wide face, her almond-round eyes narrow.

'Don't worry,' says Joe. 'I'll find someone.'

He wanders down the corridor, head craning from side to side, alert for sound and movement, alert for any sign of life. Nothing. Anna watches. Standing there, tall and dark, craned over, he looks like a big black question mark. She feels apprehensive, unsure. Joe peers into a ward. The beds are empty. No one. He scratches his head and puts his other hand in his pocket, thinking. It's like the *Marie Celeste*. Where *is* everyone?

Just then he hears the clink of kettle on cup two doors down. At last. He knocks and coughs tentatively. 'Hello?'

''Ullo there.' The nurse is standing by the sink with a cup of tea nearly at her lips. She is young, mid-30s, with blonde hair scraped back and a Brummie accent. She is trying hard to conceal her irritation at being interrupted.

'Hi, my name's Joe Gregory. My wife was told to come in tonight for a possible induction. She's expecting twins, she's done 40 weeks . . .'

'OK, hold on a minute.'

Carrying her tea, she wanders back to reception, nodding at Anna, and looks at the paperwork on the desk.

'Right, come this way.'

She walks them on to a ward, and points Anna towards a bed in an empty bay. 'Settle yourself in there,' she says.

'Um, well, Dr Fletcher assured us that we could have a side room where I could stay the night too . . .' says Joe, trying not to appear demanding.

'Out of the question, I'm afraid,' says the nurse, wandering off. 'The midwife will be along later.'

Anna undresses and gets into her nightgown. Her face is pale with tension. She is in her early 30s, but looks younger than her age. Joe prowls about by the bed. Anna flicks a book. She thinks it might make the waiting easier.

Half an hour later a midwife comes into the bay. They hear her sandals before they see her, slip-slopping along. She is small, with dark hair and a terse manner.

'I'm afraid there's nothing we can do for you this evening,' she says brusquely. 'We're short-staffed, I'm the only one around. I'm sorry but it is really nothing to do with me. If I was you, I would write to the head of midwifery and complain. The houseman will be along later, you can have a chat with him. But I don't think we will be doing anything till tomorrow.'

Joe looks at Anna. He shrugs. She pouts. They wait for the houseman.

When he comes, he is young and dapper, and has time to be friendly. He talks them through the induction process again, and apologises for messing them around. Joe feels his irritation subsiding. You have just got to get through it, he tells himself. When the houseman has gone, Joe asks Anna what she thinks he should do. Go home, she says, get a good night's sleep.

'I will ring you in the morning when they know what they are doing here,' she adds, with a smile. All the time she has her hands on her stomach, holding on to her babies. She knows only one thing: they don't want to come yet. They are happy where they are.

Anna found out she had twins at her first scan. Before she had even had a chance to look at the screen, the woman working the equipment said: 'You are aware you are expecting twins, aren't you?' Anna started laughing and looked at Joe's face. It had gone very pale.

'No,' she said, 'we had no idea.'

'Well,' said the woman, 'you are very big for twenty weeks. I thought you might have had another scan already, what with you being a twin. It is normally done earlier if there are twins in the family.'

Twins in the family. Anna has a twin sister, a fraternal twin, rather than an identical twin. But there are also identical twins on her mother's side of the family. So all in all, it was always a possibility that she would have twins. Two for the price of one, as it were.

She quite likes being a twin. Being non-identical probably makes it easier. You always have a close friend, but you have different expectations and anticipations. It is not quite the same bond as being identical – probably not the same burden. But strange things happen when you are a twin. Within weeks of Anna finding out that she was pregnant, her sister became pregnant for the first time too. She also knows that giving birth to twins can be difficult. There seem to be twice as many possible complications.

The community midwife said she could choose any hospital. Anna lived just 10 minutes' walk from St Thomas', so it made sense. She looked round the baby unit on the sixth and seventh floors of the North Wing and liked it. Parts were shabby but the staff exuded experience. They knew about twins, they dealt with all kinds of specialist births, in fact, they dealt with more births – nearly four thousand a year – than any other hospital in London. It was a specialist centre, with every kind of complication referred there: mothers with cardiac problems, diabetics, HIV-positive. They also had special twin delivery rooms, bigger than usual, with space for two medical teams, one per baby, to work. But most of all Anna liked the midwife who showed her around. She was older than the others, in her early fifties, and explained everything very simply. These are the things you use, these are the different monitors, if anything goes wrong this is what happens. The twin room is next to the operating theatre, so if they have to be delivered by Caesarean section, there is no problem. Anna's only regret was that the twin room had no view.

On her way out she looked at the low birth-weight babies, tiny creatures, barely moving, wrapped in huge nappies and cocooned in large, clear incubators. It made her feel more confident. Everyone always said that twins are premature, so she needed to feel they could cope. But maybe all that was exaggerated. When she rang her mother to ask what she thought, she said, oh, don't worry, you and your sister were 10 days late!

So Anna signed on at St Thomas'. She went to see the senior

consultant, a warm and reassuring man, who said everything would be fine, but as it was twins, they liked to do regular check-ups. So she started coming in every few weeks. Sometimes she didn't get the consultant she liked. Another doctor, a woman, told her she should stop working. Anna found her manner awkward, as if communicating with patients was the part of her job she enjoyed least. Anna didn't tell her she was going to carry on working, she didn't feel it was open to discussion. She had things she really wanted to do, and if she got tired, she reasoned, she could rest in the evening. She just smiled at the doctor and said, fine.

By the end of her pregnancy she was coming in every week, setting aside most of Thursday for the appointments. They had told her to prepare to give birth any time from 38 weeks onwards, but as the time came on, she really didn't feel that anything was going to happen. She just got bigger and bigger, and increasingly tired, but she never felt they were about to pop out. By week 40 they were talking about induction. She discussed it with Joe. They would wait one more week, then they would go along with it. Now that week is up.

Joe is still in bed when Anna rings the next morning. Nothing has happened yet, she says, so they are going to give me the first injection. Get yourself sorted out and come in afterwards, just before lunch.

Joe walks round to the hospital at midday. He finds Anna where he left her, glowering sullenly. The doctors have started the induction process with a vaginal injection of prostaglandin, just a small dose, they said, then they would see what happened. That was OK, she wanted to get on with it, but later the consultant she didn't like came round, and told her she would definitely be giving birth that afternoon. Her manner was as firm as usual, brooking no argument. Anna sighed when she left. Then nothing happened. Nothing whatsoever.

So Anna flicks her book and Joe potters around, anxiously

rearranging everything, making sure all the phone calls have been made, getting coffee, asking Anna if she is OK. Oh, stop it, she says, with a smile. Two mums come down to the ward with newborn babies, looking exhausted but happy. The staff change. Every time you build up a relationship with someone, they go off-shift, thinks Anna gloomily.

Just before four a consultant comes to talk to Anna.

'We are going to take you upstairs and break your waters,' she says, with a reassuring smile. Joe is cross, Anna feels anxious. One minute nothing is happening; the next minute you feel as if you are being rushed through at somone else's convenience. After the consultant leaves, a young midwife stops by to explain what is happening. Instantly, Joe and Anna can tell she is faintly disapproving of the whole process of induction – as if it were more for the doctor's benefit than the mother's. Anna remembers what she has heard about St Thomas' reputation for obstetricians who like to intervene, speeding things up, doing too many Caesareans. It is an old reputation, probably out of date, but these things stick. For advocates of natural childbirth, St Thomas' was, for many years, a place to be avoided.

By the time they all get upstairs, Joe and Anna are angry. They discuss who is going to say what to the next doctor they see, they feel it is all being taken out of their hands. A senior houseman appears, young and friendly, who they have met before in tow to the consultant. On his own he appears more relaxed. Joe lays into him. 'We're really angry, this is not the way we were told it would happen. One minute no one is around, next minute you are rushing us up here, breaking the waters and saying, "Get on with it!" This is no good, it's not right . . .'

'Hang on,' says the young doctor, trying to mollify him. 'There has been a misunderstanding. These drugs are intended to start opening the cervix. Once that has begun to happen, then we break the waters. From then on the drugs are redundant.' Anna sits looking at the pair of them with her hands cupped under her belly.

Joe purses his lips. Now he feels sorry for the doctor, sorry that he has flown at him.

'All right, I apologise,' he says. 'We just didn't like being told so abruptly. You know, everyone thought they would be premature, and there would be a big problem if they were, and they put a lot of onus on us to minimise that risk. We have done just about everything to minimise that risk, we got to 40 weeks and now everyone's saying, oh, we've got to get them out, we've got to get them out. We just don't need to be knocked around.'

'That's OK, I understand,' smiles the senior houseman. He is smooth and smartly dressed, confident in his charm. He can only be in his late twenties, thinks Joe, how can I trust him? He stares out of the window at the old County Hall, while the doctor chats to Anna.

'Have you thought about an epidural?' the doctor asks Anna. 'I'm not sure,' she says.

He talks to her about it and then says he will get the anaesthetist to pop in before he goes off-shift. Joe watches the river flow, under Westminster Bridge, out through the City. Maybe it's not right, he thinks, to be suspicious of doctors' motives, but you never quite know what pressures they are under, what they are trying to achieve, what they want. The action that's easiest for them might not always be best for you. Everyone knows that now. Doctors, midwives, nurses, managers – they are all accountable now, just like any other professionals. But sometimes it is hard to know who to listen to. Sometimes just finding some equilibrium, just getting through all the choices and worries, seems to be a Sisyphean task.

It is clearly going to be a long evening, he thinks, turning back to the room.

24

'It is my pleasure as chairman to welcome you all to the fourth annual general meeting of the Guy's and St Thomas' Hospital Trust . . .'

The Admiral, an upright, silver-haired pencil of a man, is standing stiffly behind a narrow temporary lectern with the G&ST logo attached. He has command of the whole parquet deck of the sumptuously panelled Governors' Hall. To his left, the Trust's senior executives sit nervously in three rows of chairs, diligently studying the new annual report or gazing at the gilded beams in the vaulted ceiling. Behind him, up on the back wall, a large white projector screen is unfurled. Beneath that, on a small raised dais, two large carved oak chairs sit like vacant thrones, one either side of a long table, as if waiting for the return of their rightful owners. The room, with its gloomy portraits hung up high – Edward VI, Florence Nightingale – and the tall, deferential cabinets of Masonic regalia outside, has a certain frosty, clandestine grandeur that fails to rub off on the executives inside. There is already a mood of tense expectation.

Facing the vacant thrones sit an audience of around 100 people, in eight rows. Many are old; most of the men are smartly dressed in suits and ties, the women in sensible skirts and coats. Among them are a sprinkling of concerned professionals – health authority executives, community health council representatives – and one MP, Simon Hughes, whose constituency contains Guy's. Everyone has an axe to grind. The evening meeting is the only chance the general public have to question the Trust's executives on strategy and policy. At the back of the room Matt Tee sits quietly next to a table of brochures and releases, chatting to a journalist. He is nodding and whispering. 'The Princess Diana Victims of War Memorial Hospital,' he says, 'but we are not leaking it yet. It is just at the idea stage.'

The Admiral clicks a switch on an infra-red hand unit by the lectern, and a new slide is thrown up on the screen behind him: his name and title. He makes a brief introduction, highlighting two significant events from the year: the opening of the new hospital building at Guy's, and the Trust's initiatives to get closer to patients in the community. His tone is firm, if a little stiff. The audience look stonily on. The idea behind the meeting is that, just as quoted company boards give their shareholders a chance every year to hear what they are doing and put questions, so a Trust's 'shareholders' – patients, staff and other professionals – must see that the hospital's bosses are accountable for their actions. When those actions include the implementation of a highly controversial merger of two famous old hospitals, the potential for discord is large.

Finally the Admiral introduces the chief executive, who stands up, looking uncharacteristically severe in a dark blue suit and tie, and grasps the infra-red handset. Within a few seconds he is muttering and crouching like a schoolboy with a remote-control car, trying to make it work. A few glances are exchanged in the audience until, finally, with a definitive click, the slide changes and his name is up in lights.

His presentation is brief. He runs through the in-patient figures for the Trust: 22,900 day cases seen, down from 24,200 the year before; 21,300 elective cases, down from 23,900. The Trust could do more work, he explains, but local health authorities simply don't have the cash to buy the operations they need. He continues: 33,300 emergency admissions, up from 31,900 two years previously; 160,000 attending A&E on both sites, up from 144,000 two years previously; and births slightly down, at 7,800. In the last three years, he says, the number of non-emergency patients treated by the Trust has fallen by 7 per cent, while the number of those on the waiting list for operations has increased by 28 per cent. An increasing number of patients are having to wait the maximum 18 months.

He points out that, nevertheless, the Trust's financial performance is strong. Next week, he adds, it will present its business case to the Department of Health for a new women and children's hospital to be built on the St Thomas' site. It will be unique in London, bringing together the full range of services for women and children. No other centre, not even Great Ormond Street Hospital, will match it. He expects a response within three months. If approved, the work can start next year, the 50th anniversary of the National Health Service. The outlook has to be good, he concludes. He then introduces the new medical director, a St Thomas' radiologist, who, he says, will make his own presentation before introducing two of his colleagues. They too will make presentations. There is some shuffling of feet among the audience, who know full well that every word said eats into the two hours running time habitually allocated for the AGM. The Admiral likes to wrap it up well before 8 p.m. The equations seem simple to some: more presentations, fewer questions, though that is probably a harsh judgement.

The new medical director is blond and boyish, and looks ten years younger than his age. He starts tentatively with a bad joke about the spelling of his name, and then runs through his CV. Qualified at Bart's in 1966. Became a consultant at St Thomas' in 1975. 'I am pleased to join the executive board after a time of politics, siteism . . .' A few heads go up in the audience, who until now have been steadfastedly examining the annual report's figures. '. . . and I am looking forward to bringing the focus back on to clinical care.' He discusses the 'critical mass of activity', links with GPs and the aims for a 'seamless service'. He emphasises how concerned he is with the increase in waiting lists, and hands over to the next speaker, the clinical director in charge of dietetics. She, after describing at length what her department does, hands over to the head of cancer services who, after explaining in detail how Britain's cancer services have developed, and how his department is linking up with King's to become a designated cancer centre for London, hands back to the chairman. It is over an hour since the AGM began. A ripple of anticipation – straightened backs and cleared throats – runs through the audience.

'OK, I will take questions from the audience now,' says the Admiral, peering over his half-moon glasses at the forest of hands that are instantly upstretched. He gazes round the audience. He is not expecting any plaudits. Matt Tee sent a memo round earlier, warning executives about the sort of questions they could expect: how many operations cancelled, how many complaints, why are you spending money on new buildings at St Thomas' when parts of Guy's stand empty, why will you not expand ITU when cardiac patients are dying because they can't have operations, why – if you made a surplus last year – aren't you paying staff more or keeping more beds open? No one had any illusions about the reception they were likely to get. The campaign to Save Guy's may not have been as high-profile as that fighting the closure of Bart's across the river, which ran a weekly demonstration, but it was well organised and had wide support outside the hospital (probably more so than inside, where only four consultants publicly backed it). At every AGM it pulled itself together like Charles I's old cavalry for one more charge at the Roundheads.

'Yes, sir, you in the middle . . .'

A confident man in shirt and slacks stands up. His tone is subtly snide. 'I am the chair of Southwark Community Health Council. This evening I have heard that day cases and elective cases are down, yet new facilities are being built for day and elective cases. I have also heard that the number of cases in A&E is up and yet Guy's A&E is being downgraded to a minor injuries department. May I humbly put forward, sir, that this suggests that the Trust's strategy has taken place in spite of, rather than because of, the figures?'

The chairman, holding his lectern with both hands, smiles tensely and passes the question over to Matthews. He stands, one hand in his pocket, and searches for the right words. 'As far as, erm ... day cases are, erm ... concerned ...' The whole point of putting elective work on to the Guy's site and moving acute services out, he says, was so that operations wouldn't have to be cancelled because of emergencies, thus extending waiting lists further. 'As far as A&E is concerned I can only repeat what I said in my presentation: that the volume of demand is properly met by the ...'

As he finishes, at least 20 hands are already up, reaching towards the beamed ceiling, as their owners crane to make eye contact with the Admiral. When the chief executive finishes, the Admiral points to a tall old man at the back, wearing a charcoal suit and a services tie. He stands up very slowly, clutching a wad of hand-written notes. He gives his name, speaking in a tight, upper-class accent that seems eerily out of place with the proceedings, and runs through his credentials.

'I am a member of the Save Guy's committee, a patient representative, and I have been a voluntary worker at Guy's for sixteen years. Now we have all heard about the lack of money currently in the NHS, and I am greatly concerned about it, yet we hear from you today that money is being found instead of PFI to provide new buildings and resources at St Thomas' in place of those that exist at Guy's. The latter are currently situated at a public transport hub. They are used by patients who come in from Kent and south-east London. These patients will have to come past London Bridge to reach St Thomas'. This further extension of their journey time is as unwelcome as it is inconvenient. St Thomas' is relatively isolated in terms of public transport. It seems to me that it is complete folly to persist with the present Trust strategy!' A mutter of approval and a short spatter of applause runs across the audience.

'I also see,' he goes on, 'that the Trust has sanctioned the claim that it is not closing Guy's. This is a half-truth. The new Thomas Guy House is being dedicated to a 120-bed orthopaedic set-up. There will be a day-care centre and a mass of out-patient clinics. That is fine for people who are served by these specialities, but for most people locally it means nothing at all. What you are closing is practically everything that they have come to rely upon from Guy's over the last 200 years!'

The Admiral interjects quickly: 'Well, thank you for that lengthy and detailed question. I would repeat the statement we made earlier, that we are not closing Guy's. The vast majority of our patients *are* out-patients, and the same number will be going through as go through today. I would stress again that the arguments are about the drawing together of the clinical strengths and the advantages of concentrating elective work. It is unforgivable that we are in a position on both sites where patients are booked in for planned operations and are then cancelled because of emergencies.'

The Admiral looks across at the chief executive, sitting with the board, deeply immersed in the annual report on his lap. 'Do you want to add anything, Tim?'

'Er, no,' smiles Matthews, his gaze fixed upon the portrait of Edward VI. He wouldn't be human if he wasn't thinking: *four years after the Government rubber-stamped the merger strategy, and they are still arguing this one out interminably. Extraordinary. Why do these people think that one institution has to be throttled for the other to thrive?*

Because, perhaps, that is what it looks like.

25

Anna is twisted in the bath, her back arched in pain, her limbs dwarfed by her hugely protuberant belly. She feels no contractions, just pain, like a mix of stomach cramps and a knife in the kidneys, twisting slowly, never stopping, never ebbing and flowing, just constantly there. Joe doesn't know what to do. After all the fuss about breaking Anna's waters, the doctors never did it. They checked her cervix, found it hadn't dilated at all, and gave her another injection. Joe stayed to talk to the anaesthetist, who had reassured them about the epidural, but warned Anna that it would be difficult to walk around once the line was in. Joe liked the anaesthetist – he looked like the kind of man who probably played flanker in the hospital rugby team, tough and fast. He was prepared to talk everything through in a down-to-earth manner. Anna felt she had been given all the information to make the right choice. It put her in a good mood. She sent Joe home for an hour. 'Nothing is going to happen yet,' she said, 'check the messages.' Then the pain kicked in. By the time Joe got back, Anna was in agony, trying to soothe her torment in a hot bath.

A midwife comes in with a painkiller and a sleeping pill. Don't worry, she says, the pain is good, it must mean something is going to happen. Just hang on in there. She tells Anna and Joe they can stay in the delivery suite anteroom, unless things get too busy. The quiet is eerie. Either the other delivery rooms are empty or just very well soundproofed. Once only, when Joe leaves Anna to get a drink of water, does he think he hears a moan, just softly, as if from someone under torture in a basement far away, then it goes again. Maybe it's a slack evening. He remembers the midwife telling them about seasonal patterns and inexplicable factors, like full moons and local high tides, when there are always more births. Maybe the Thames is low tonight. He wonders if he can tell from his window.

Later Anna lies on the bed, holding Joe's hand. The sleeping pill and painkiller are soothing her now. Joe sits up next to her on a couple of chairs pushed together. He feels the grip of Anna's hand loosening as she drifts off to sleep.

Then Anna sits upright and screams loudly, a cry of sudden deep anguish. Joe leaps up with a start and rings the bell for the midwife. The pain, says Anna, it is so intense.

'I'm going to be sick, I'm going to be sick,' she shouts. Joe finds a cardboard carton, then, worrying that that won't be big enough, runs for the wastepaper bin. Anna starts retching over it. Later she remembers being sick everywhere but nothing comes out.

The midwife bustles in. She is broad and West Indian, calm and competent. She asks what is the matter, and tells Anna to lie down so she can examine her cervix. Two centimetres dilated. It's started.

The midwife goes out for a minute then returns with gas for Anna to breathe. Gas and air. Take it, she says, take it. Anna screams again. Then she takes the gas. She screams, then she takes the gas again.

'Take the gas,' says the midwife.

'I am!' shouts Anna. 'You don't mind me screaming, do you?' she asks Joe.

'If it makes you feel better, love, scream as loudly as you can.' He is rubbing her back now, trying to soothe her. She is off the bed, walking half-crouched round the room, pausing only to take quick shots of the gas before screaming again.

'Jaargggh!'

The midwife lies her down again and checks the dilation. The cervix is opening rapidly. Yet still Anna is not feeling any contractions, just prolonged pain. She sits up on the bed, panting and shuddering.

The midwife waits for a lull and then says: 'We have got to get you next door and get the epidural in.'

Anna nods sweatily.

'It's going to be OK,' says Joe, 'it's going to be OK.'

26

The hands fly up again.

'You, sir,' says the Admiral, 'on the left.'

An angular middle-aged man, wearing a crumpled suit and tie, rises, hands clutching notes.

'I am a director of the Save Guy's campaign. I have a series of linked questions.'

A light wince passes over the Admiral's face.

'Go on,' he says with cold courtesy.

'First, what are the estimated capital costs of the new building at St Thomas'? Second, will the new business plan for the building be published? Third, will you confirm that the capital cost of Thomas Guy House is £160m? Fourth, what is projected for premises that have been vacated on the Guy's site? Fifth, what specialities are to remain at Guy's? Sixth, what does the Trust plan to do if public money is not forthcoming for the development? Seventh, what are the number of elective beds projected for this site and for Guy's? Eighth, does the Trust have cognisance of the latest research on optimum hospital size and the benefits derived therefrom?'

The man sits down. The Admiral sighs. He is still writing furiously on a pad. 'I think I have got all that down,' he says, rather testily. Then he looks up. 'Right, question one, the projected cost of the women and children's hospital at St Thomas' is £114m. Two, the business plan is not a document we will publish, but if you wish to view it I am sure we could let you read it in the office. Three, the cost of Thomas Guy House will be around £160m. As to the use of premises . . .'

The Admiral, looking his questioner straight in the eye,

launches into a lengthy description of the possible alternative uses for parts of the Guy's site. His tone is icy, his delivery slow and methodical. He works his way through the questions. By the time he reaches the number of beds, an inquisitive hush has settled on the room. '. . . And beds?' The Admiral looks at the new medical director for support. The medical director tells him the projected figures. 'Nine hundred and eighty-one beds on this site and, ah, 153 on the Guy's site, plus 56 mental health beds.'

There is a stunned silence while the audience takes in the significance of the figures. Five times as many beds at St Thomas'. The figures have been in public circulation for some time, but just to hear them out loud seems to confirm the audience's worst fears.

'As to optimum hospital sizes . . .' the Admiral is really earning his crust, fluently batting the questions. 'Ah, yes, the principal of the medical school, you haven't said much yet.'

There is an edge of antagonism to his comment. The principal looks up sharply, and waves the suggestion away, saying he doesn't know the area. Matthews smiles, and asks loudly, 'May I?'

'Of course,' says the Admiral.

'There is research available to show just about anything you want, that big is better or that small is the best,' says Matthews confidently. But, he adds, people shouldn't assume that just because St Thomas' has all the beds it is going to be a much livelier site. The majority of 'traffic' in hospitals is out-patients and investigative work. With much of that removed to Guy's, the St Thomas' site will actually seem rather quiet.

'Next question?' asks the Admiral, raising his bushy grey eyebrows. 'You, madam,' pointing to a young woman in a blue blazer near the front. She sits up straight before making her first point.

'First of all I would like the board to comment on the fact that it plans to spend £114m of public money on a super-building when it has already spent £160m on an out-patients' block. Then I would like . . .'

The Admiral scribbles while she runs through her list. They are not so much questions as accusations. At one point she pauses, and the Admiral interjects: 'Can you just repeat your first three questions, then you can have your eight, if eight you must have.'

The woman sucks her cheeks in, suddenly red with anger. She looks as if she is making a large effort to control her fury.

'It would be nice,' she snaps, 'if you could admit that the way in which the money was used for Thomas Guy House was a disgrace!'

The Admiral sighs again. 'Any building that has been built for a specific purpose is out of date 20 years later. The fact that Thomas Guy House was 15 years in gestation . . .'

'No!' shouts a man at the side. There is a low murmur of agitation from the audience. It is clear that the board has few sympathisers.

'Look,' says the Admiral, 'I am trying to address the question. I am trying not to be rude to you.' He pauses. 'Buildings have to be adaptable, things do vary over the years.'

The woman bristles back. 'But what about the waiting times at St Thomas' A&E?'

The chairman turns to the nursing director, a broad Scotswoman sitting at the back. 'Well,' she says. 'Patients are seen immediately on arrival in A&E. The serious cases are then seen immediately . . .'

There is agitated shuffling in the audience as they realise she is busking.

'What I am asking for,' says the questioner, half shouting now, 'is proper figures for how long people are waiting, and I am amazed you don't have them . . .'

'Right,' the Admiral cuts in, 'I am sorry the director of A&E is not here this evening, as I am sure he would have the figures.'

The woman scowls. There is a tense silence. She continues: 'I am very pleased that the Trust has now accepted that co-operation and not confrontation is the best way forward. I would like to hear you say that publicly you have changed your policy.'

The Admiral's fixed smile never wavers. Co-operation, he says, has always been the board's policy. 'Next question?'

A young man in a suit stands up. 'I am sure we were given an earlier figure of £151m for the new building project at St Thomas'. It doesn't really give you a great deal of confidence in the board if changes are made all the time.'

'Well,' says the Admiral, peering over his spectacles, 'different figures are right at different times with different scenarios.'

'The figure that interests me,' says the next questioner, 'is the chief executive's £116,000 salary. A large element in his increase from last year's figure is a performance-related bonus. That will come as something of a surprise to many who work in the Trust, after what has happened here. It also probably hasn't occurred to the non-executive directors on the board that by increasing the chief executive's salary, it makes it much more difficult for him to get another job.'

A little laugh rolls round the room. Matthews looks steadfastly down at the annual report on his lap while his fellow board members shift uneasily in their seats.

'Well, I don't quite know how to answer that,' says the Admiral, returning the questioner's stare. 'He is not the highest-paid chief executive in London, and it has been a very busy year . . .'

27

'JAAAARRGGGGH! JEEEAAARRGGGGH!'

Anna is up on the bed in the twins delivery suite. Suddenly the room is full of people: senior midwife, junior midwife, student

midwife, senior houseman, senior obstetric registrar, paediatrician, anaesthetist. Joe recognises some of them; others are
strangers. They hover around, adjusting their gowns, preparing
the two little resuscitation tables and sorting out the tubes and
bottles under the bright strip lights. The anaesthetist sets up the
epidural into the small of Anna's back. As the drugs wash in she
feels the pain subside slightly.

They have broken her waters. She is 10cm dilated now. The
midwives cluster round, encouraging her, exhorting her, soothing
her. Joe stays by her head, whispering in her ear. The doctors
monitor the babies' heart rates. There are signs of distress, they
want to get them out fast. Anna is numb below the waist now.
She doesn't even feel the episiotomy. She knows they have done
it because the midwives keep asking Joe, 'Are you all right?' They
think he is going to faint. Anna keeps pushing but she feels she
isn't getting anywhere.

'I'm going to use the suction cup,' says the registrar. He gently
inserts the squished yellow head of the cup into Anna, searching
for the babies' head. Joe waits tensely.

'What's that?' asks Joe.

A gentler way of helping the baby out than using forceps,
explains the registrar, working fast. Once inside, the suction
cup re-forms around the baby's head, and is gently attached
by use of a vacuum pump. Then the baby can be guided out.
Joe makes a face.

'Are you all right?' asks a midwife again.

'Yeah, fine, fine.'

'Come on, push!'

Anna's face is contorted into an anguished rictus.

A shout goes up. 'The baby's coming . . .'

'Come on, Anna, nearly there.'

'Here we go . . .'

The crown of the baby, capped in the cup, then the face very
slowly emerges, as if Anna's body is unwilling to let go. Then
suddenly, as the shoulders emerge, the rest of the baby's body

slithers slipperily out, patches of white skin just visible through the yellow, blue and black mucus.

'Yes!'

'It's a girl,' shouts the midwife, quickly cutting the umbilical cord.

Anna is up on her elbows, her face contorted. Joe can see the widening pool of blood on the sheets. She is losing too much blood, he thinks. The paediatrician walks the baby to the resuscitation table. His team work quickly, cleaning her up, sucking off the meconium, wrapping her in a blanket. Joe leaves Anna's side to look at the baby. She is small, 2.8kg in weight, but long and beautiful, with delicate fair hair and a pug face. Joe strokes her hand, little bigger than his right thumb. He marvels over the little fingernails, tiny millimetres of hardening flesh. The midwife whisks up the baby to show to Anna. She holds her close, so Anna can see without her glasses.

'You have got a beautiful daughter, Anna.'

'Come on, one more to go.'

The paediatrician hovers over the monitors and Joe feels a tight air of tension descend on the room. The doctors are exchanging looks, not saying much.

'What's happening? What's going on?' asks Joe.

'She is going to be all right,' says the midwife.

'Don't worry,' says one of the doctors, 'we're going to sort it out. It looks like the second baby is very distressed. We need to get the baby out.'

Anna is exhausted and weak. The team work fast, inserting a monitor on the baby's head inside her. They look at the readings without emotion, giving nothing away. Joe watches anxiously. Another suction cup is inserted in an attempt to pull the second baby out. It doesn't work. The doctors are cursing; the sealant between the vacuum pump and the cup has broken. The registrar struggles in vain to tape up the leak.

'Forceps,' he says quietly.

Joe is rubbing Anna's back again. 'It's going to be all right,' he repeats, 'it's going to be all right.' Nothing will go wrong, he tells himself. If they can't get the baby out, they can do a Caesarean. It's still OK. He feels torn between comforting Anna and watching over his new daughter. She has been abandoned on one side of the room as everyone concentrates on the next baby.

It is half an hour since the first baby came out and still the team are working.

'OK, I think I've got it.'

The second baby slides out, smaller than the first, emaciated, with flipper hands and feet and a large head.

'It's a boy . . .'

The medical team quickly cut the umbilical cord and whisk the baby away to the resuscitation table. Anna sits up again and strains to see across the corner of the room. Everyone is standing round the table. Without her glasses, it is just a blur. Anna has tears rolling down her face. She cannot see the expression on Joe's face, she cannot see what the team are doing, she just hears the paediatrician's instructions.

'Suck here, and here! COME ON! Oxygen mask!'

My baby is dead, she thinks, my baby is dead. I know he is dead.

28

Next question. 'I am a GP,' says a nervous woman in row five, twisting her fingers as she speaks, 'and I want to point out that there is great concern among GPs about the closure of Guy's A&E. The chief executive wrote to the chairman of our GP group recently and asked for a letter of support for the closure plan, and we felt we couldn't give it. Now, there are 42 GPs in my group, and we are very concerned about what is going to happen.'

'Can I answer that?' A tall, anxious man in a slightly dishevelled suit, sitting just in front of the questioner, gets to his feet. 'I am chief executive of the health authority. We have to take a strategic view of the whole area. We have approved a policy of concentrating resources at three A&Es: King's, Lewisham and St Thomas'. There would be more people unhappy if we didn't follow the policy through.' It has been worked through, he goes on, with the London Ambulance Service, and will produce a string of benefits.

Eventually the Admiral turns to Simon Hughes, who has been waiting patiently at the side of the room for his turn to speak. He stands slowly, brushing his hand over his hair, which is swept across a bald patch at the back of his head. He is wearing a blue blazer, white shirt and striped tie, and is clutching a pad of notes. None of the board has any illusions about what he will ask. Since Guy's is in his constituency, he has felt publicly bound to support the local Save Guy's campaign, even if privately he will often acknowledge that the merger plans make sense. His knack for the public gesture is not always appreciated by the Trust's senior executives.

'I want to apologise for being late,' he starts, 'but I would ask the Trust again if they could possibly desist from organising their annual general meetings during party political conferences . . .'

'We have tried to do this,' says the Admiral curtly, and not totally convincingly, 'but I am afraid it is bound up with when we have to publish the figures.'

'Well, there are a few points I would like to make first. Overall, I think most people in my constituency are opposed to the strategy that the Trust is following. Patients, residents and users just don't seem to be any happier than they were last year. I would love them to be, because I am a big fan of the NHS and there is a lot of good work which goes on here, but I think that most people hope that next year there will be a different strategy.

'Now, I have some questions. First, will you give a commitment that orthopaedic trauma won't move early from Guy's, as that would undermine A&E work there? Second, I don't understand a strategy that has elective beds at Guy's but keeps some elective beds at St Thomas', and has out-patients at Guy's, and keeps some out-patients at St Thomas'. It seems to me that St Thomas' is getting a huge block of all the work. The effect will be that Guy's specialists and students will see that there is very little work for them there, and they will all want to go to St Thomas'. Third, why should the NHS pay a penny for a new building when you can put the same women and children's services in a building they have already got at Guy's? Some of us will need a lot of persuading that Thomas Guy House should not be used to the full. It was, after all, built for in-patient use. Fourthly, why are there so many complaints about the services offered by the Trust? I want to know what the strategy for complaints is . . .'

'All right,' says the Admiral, 'let's start with . . .'

'I haven't finished yet,' says Hughes tersely.

'Look,' says the Admiral, hardening his tone, 'you are not in the House now.'

29

Joe is leaning over Anna, whispering in her ear. 'It's OK, he is going to be OK, don't worry.'

The paediatrician comes across. 'I think he is going to be fine. Try not to worry. We have got to sort you out next.'

He tells Joe he is just going to see if he can get the boy a bed in neo-natal intensive care. Joe walks back to look at his babies, so small. The boy is just 2.2kg. His face looks pinched and thin, his lips tight, as if he is pursing them all the time. The skin round his neck hangs in loose folds. He seems weak and quiet.

Joe turns to Anna but she is surrounded by doctors and

midwives. He hears just snatches of conversation ... placenta not coming ... have to take her to theatre ... more epidural ... is theatre free? Then Anna's voice: what will happen if they don't come? Matter-of-fact response: you will be poisoned. Suddenly they are wheeling her off.

'Where are you going?' says Joe.

'We're going to have to take the placentas out with forceps. We'll do it in the operating theatre. You stay here,' says the senior houseman. The placentas, which have nourished the babies for so long, carrying food and oxygen from the bloodstream, are now threatening Anna. Joe grabs Anna's hand. 'It will be OK,' he says, 'I know it will.' She squeezes back.

The paediatrician checks the boy again. 'I think he is going to be fine,' he repeats, almost as if he is trying to convince himself. The boy's blood oxygen level has gone up from 6.8 to 7.2, a good sign, he tells Joe. A midwife wraps the boy up tight and gives him to Joe to hold. Then she passes him a bottle and says, 'Feed him.'

Joe gives her a puzzled, frightened look. She shows him how to hold the baby, how to nuzzle his lips with the bottle. Soon the lips open and the baby starts feeding voraciously. Another good sign, says the midwife. He wants to live.

30

'And can I make a final point?' asks Hughes, gazing round the audience for support, leaving a little pregnant pause before the final barbed assault. 'If the strategy is changed, will you all work as enthusiastically for a new strategy?'

The Admiral's eyes narrow. Matthews looks at his feet. 'I will remind you that I and my board are government employees and will follow government policy,' says the Admiral, with icy formality, 'and I resent any suggestion that we won't.'

He runs through some answers to Hughes' points. 'Now, complaints, we had 600,000 patients through these doors last year. From that we got 800 written complaints. I see just the tip of the iceberg, the ones that rise to the top. I spend the majority of my day dealing with these complaints and I assure you we take them seriously. Now, I will ask our director of quality and nursing to tell you what we are doing about them.'

'Firstly,' she says, 'may I say that we are aware that this is an area where we have got to improve, and can I apologise for the distress this has caused any of our patients . . .' She runs through the complaints procedure.

The chairman of the local community health council stands up to interrupt her. 'I think the Trust needs to have a fundamental review of the way the complaints system works. I know people are trying their best, and most of those I deal with are very good about it, but it is not working.'

The board avoids eye contact. The next questioner recounts a long anecdote about a woman who nearly died from an aneurism but was saved by the fact that she lived near Guy's A&E. If the ambulance had had to take her to St Thomas' she would be dead. Then another smartly dressed old man stands up and introduces himself as the chairman of the Friends of Guy's Hospital. 'The Friends,' he says, 'are very loyal to the hospital and do not feel they are getting a good deal. I look at this august panel, sir,' he runs his hand through the air, gesturing at the board sitting in front of him, 'and I do not see many who would have a deep understanding of the history of Guy's Hospital. Anyway, to the point. The Friends supply a lot of things for the hospital. We are thinking of supplying curtains for all the beds in New Guy's House. It is going to cost us a great deal of money. Can you promise that you are going to be there for six or seven years and not going to pull a fast one?'

The Admiral assures him there are no plans to pull out of that part of the Guy's site in the immediate future, and says he is welcome to check any spending plans with the board at any time. 'Time for one more question, I think.'

'Sir!'

The director of the Save Guy's campaign stands up again.

'Oh, come on,' says the Admiral, 'you have had your eight questions.'

31

Anna feels nothing. She is lying in the operating theatre, numbed and exhausted. She can see them working feverishly to extract the placentas from her womb. She is shunted and tugged and pulled, but she is so weak and exhausted she does not resist.

'I want to see it,' she says, finally.

'Really?'

'Really.'

The doctor walks round with a plastic kidney dish. Inside, the placenta looks like a piece of blue-black liver. She nods. She just wanted to know.

Joe is taken to another room across the corridor from the delivery suite. An incubator is wheeled in. The boy is placed inside and Joe holds the little girl. 'Is Anna going to be OK?' he asks one of the doctors.

'Yeah, I think so,' he says, scratching his head. Suddenly he looks very young. The whole team are young, thinks Joe, only the senior midwife is older than me.

'She's lost a lot of blood and she is pretty tired, but we'll put her back together again.' The doctor grins sheepishly.

'Can she breast-feed?' asks Joe.

'I'll leave that to the midwives,' says the doctor. 'They'll be here in a second.'

A couple of minutes after he has left, Anna is wheeled in. She is nearly unconscious with exhaustion, but she is clean and stitched and dressed. She can barely talk, and everyone else is speaking at once. Joe is dazed. He makes out that she will need a blood transfusion.

'Everything is going to be fine,' says the midwife.

Later the paediatrician comes back and explains everything to Joe. If it's a difficult delivery it is quite normal for the second twin to be distressed, and when they are underweight as well, they start taking energy from where they can, which is why they take oxygen out of the blood, which is why the blood oxygen level was low, and why they worked fast to re-oxygenate him. The details blur but Joe sees now how much the paediatrician anticipated, how much the whole team knew what was probably coming, but didn't let on.

Then the senior houseman joins them. He is quite open about it: that was a bad one, he says, it's not surprising Anna is a bit knocked about, I mean, there were five different major complications. Induced labour, forceps delivery, manual retrieval of the placenta . . . Joe loses count. He can see how relieved the doctor is, but also exhilarated. Of course, the team are on a high, he thinks, as if they have just played a brilliant game of football or created some momentous artwork, against all the odds, snatching victory from the jaws of defeat. They want to go over it all, they want to live it again, and why not? They deserve every bit of praise he can give them. They never panicked. In fact, the only impression he got was that it would take a lot more to shake either them or the midwives. Nothing was too tough. If they set their shoulder to the rock and pushed hard enough, they could get it over the hill. For good.

A week later Anna and her babies go home. They are fine.

32

'It's a statement, not a question, OK?'

'All right,' sighs the Admiral.

'Yes, right, to sum up, I feel there is an undercurrent of serious dissatisfaction here. There is a bias towards St Thomas' in this Trust which is unfair and we feel should be corrected!' A loud cheer goes up from the audience. The Admiral looks on, unmoved. He waits for the noise to die down before replying.

'Well, I don't doubt that there is a considerable body of support for the Save Guy's campaign here tonight, but we have a strategy that has been approved by the Department of Health and we will stick to it. It is not pro-Thomas' or anti-Guy's, or anti-Guy's history. We have got to take the best of both institutions and build on that. OK, I am drawing the meeting to a close now. I would like to thank you all for coming. Thank you.'

As the meeting winds up, the audience file out in knots and the board members stand together and cluster, smiling nervously. Another year gone, they seem to sigh. Tee joins them, making reassuring noises. The Admiral busies himself at the lectern, pushing his papers together. Matthews sits pensively, bottom lip over top, smiling faintly, his eyes featureless behind wide glasses, his thoughts unreadable. If he is wondering whether this is any way to run a hospital, with so much acrimony and doubt imposed from outside, he doesn't show it. He knows that everybody is right. The NHS needs a long-term plan for London, rather than piecemeal development, and that plan must include some concentration of hospital resources. Equally, you would be a fool not to fight in order to preserve those resources at the hospital you love, especially when primary care is so poor. For patients, the Trust's financial success is immaterial if the services don't match up to expectation. And expectations get higher every year.

Some things never change. There are no easy answers. Matthews sits still, staring straight ahead. To an onlooker, he has the slightly dazed, resigned look of a man who keeps walking into walls.

33

Over in A&E, a young man, drunk, sobs over the unconscious body of his younger brother, lying on a trolley in Resus. Both have been out on a drinking bender, during which the younger brother slipped and knocked himself out, gashing his head badly. He has been lying in the cubicle for half an hour, while the doctors work to ascertain just how bad his injuries are. His brother, uncertain and dazed, crouches by him, fiddling with the height-control cog on the side of the trolley-bed, looking as if he is about to wheel his brother away. A nurse, catching his actions as she walks past, asks him to leave.

'Fock off! He's my brother!' the young man screams. 'FOCK OFF! I'M STAYING!'

The nurse stares him down.

'I said OUT!' she snaps, and for a moment they meet, nose to nose, breath on breath. The man's face puckers in rage before he sways slightly and retreats. The nurse ushers him off to reception with disdainful determination.

There, amid the day's debris of crisp packets and Coke cans, he slouches in front of the television, murmuring agitatedly to himself. The room is nearly empty. Only a mother waits with her child, red-faced and tearful. Two ambulancemen chat up the receptionist. A cleaner tidies round them. Outside, the rush-hour traffic is just beginning to subside, and the first patter of dark raindrops sweeps the dirty streets.

February 1998. The Labour government, after establishing a review of strategy for London's hospitals, declined to fund the plans drawn up by the Guy's and St Thomas' Trust for a new women and children's hospital on the St Thomas' site. Instead, it asked the Trust to look again at making better use of the facilities at Guy's. The government did, however, approve the proposal to shut Guy's A&E department. The Trust responded by announcing that it would build a smaller hospital for children at St Thomas', funded by £37m from the Special Trustees. At time of writing, there is no intention to name it after Diana, Princess of Wales. The Trust also declared that it would now base its cancer and renal services at Guy's, raising the planned number of beds on the site to 250, and launched an appeal for funds to build a new Sexual Health Institute in the South Wing on the St Thomas' site. The Institute would bring together outpatient, academic and research facilities, and co-ordinate the treatment of patients with HIV and AIDS.

ACKNOWLEDGEMENTS

This book would not have been possible without the enthusiastic cooperation of many of those working at St Thomas' Hospital. Some who helped me, for reasons of discretion, asked not to be named and I respect their wishes. I am, however, deeply grateful to every doctor, nurse, student, manager and staff member at the hospital, from the chief executive and medical director down, who generously gave me interview time, and more than that, put up with me shadowing them, watching them work and badgering them with questions. I have nothing but the deepest admiration and respect for the manner in which many of them carry out their work under pressures which in other professions would be deemed intolerable. I am also grateful to all the patients who gave me permission to write about their treatment and who faithfully told me their stories, and to those outside the hospital who offered me advice, sent me books and read my drafts. Finally, I would like to thank Richard Beswick and Antonia Hodgson at Little, Brown for their input, and Vanessa Nicolson, Elena Davidson and Rosa Davidson for their love and encouragement. Like Robert Bruce's spider, we never give up.

This book is also dedicated to the memory of an old friend, Oscar Moore, who I miss, and who would have enjoyed the struggle.

EARTH ODYSSEY

Mark Hertsgaard

'If you want to understand the next century as it unfolds,
this is the required background reading'
Bill McKibben, author of *The End of Nature*

Like many of us, Mark Hertsgaard has long worried about
the declining health of our environment. But in 1991, he
decided to act on his concern and investigate the escalating
crisis for himself. He embarked on an odyssey lasting most
of the decade and spanning 19 countries. Now, in *Earth
Odyssey*, he reports on our environmental predicament
through the eyes of the people who live it.

From the gilded boardrooms of Paris to the traffic-clogged
streets of Bangkok, we travel from the deep human past to
our still unfolding future. Much of the story revolves around
people like Zhenbing, Hertsgaard's charismatic interpreter in
China, whose desire to escape poverty leaves him indifferent
to his country's horrific air and water pollution. Drawing on
interviews with Vaclav Havel, Al Gore, Jacques Cousteau,
and numerous other prominent figures, Hertsgaard offers
fresh insight into such complex issues as humanity's growing
addiction to the automobile, the insidious spread of nuclear
technology, and the inevitable tension between unfettered
capitalism and the health of the biosphere.

Combining first-rate reportage with irresistible story-telling,
Mark Hertsgaard has written an essential – and ultimately
hopeful – book about the uncertain fate of humankind.

Abacus
0 349 11181 2

THE ENCYCLOPAEDIA OF PSYCHOACTIVE SUBSTANCES

Richard Rudgley

'Fascinating . . . Suddenly, clubland seems tame' *Esquire*

From chocolate to cocaine, glue sniffing to giraffe liver, LSD to lettuce, *The Encyclopaedia of Psychoactive Substances* provides the first reliable, comprehensive exploration of one of the most misunderstood, widespread and ancient human activities – the chemical quest for altered states of consciousness.

'Formidable . . . Rudgley's curiosity, distilled concentration, inter-disciplinary connectiveness, deadpan humour, prodigious reading, magpie eclecticism and anecdotal ease are all massively appealing'
Jonathan Meades, *Evening Standard*

'Startling' *Guardian*

'Complete and authoritative . . . excellent . . . fascinating'
Loaded

'This really is a fun read . . . there are great little bits of information, such as the one about Eton schoolboys being flogged in the 17th century if they *forgot* to bring their tobacco pipes to school' Will Self, *New Statesman*

'Will deeply satisfy the curious . . . impressive'
Nicholas Lezard, *Modern Review*

'A thorough and entertaining reference text' *New Scientist*

Abacus
0 349 11127 8

Now you can order superb titles directly from Abacus

☐	Earth Odyssey	Mark Hertsgaard	£9.99
☐	The Encyclopaedia of Psychoactive Substances	Richard Rudgley	£8.99

―――――――――――― (ABACUS) ――――――――――――

Please allow for postage and packing: **Free UK delivery.**
Europe; add 25% of retail price; Rest of World; 45% of retail price.

To order any of the above or any other Abacus titles, please call our
credit card orderline or fill in this coupon and send/fax it to:

Abacus, 250 Western Avenue, London, W3 6XZ, UK.
Fax 0181 324 5678   Telephone 0181 324 5517

☐ I enclose a UK bank cheque made payable to Abacus for £...........

☐ Please charge £........... to my Access, Visa, Delta, Switch Card No.

☐☐☐☐☐☐☐☐☐☐☐☐☐☐☐☐☐☐☐

Expiry date ☐☐☐☐   Switch Issue No. ☐☐

Name (Block Letters please) _____

Address _____

_____

_____

Post/zip code:_____   Telephone _____

Signature _____

Please allow 28 days for delivery within the UK. Offer subject to price and availability.
Please do not send any further mailings from companies carefully selected by Abacus ☐